BMA

BMA Library

Sixth Edition

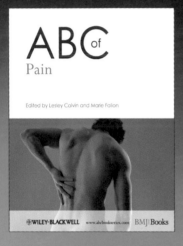
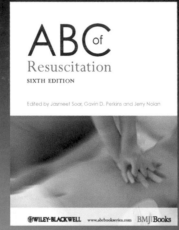
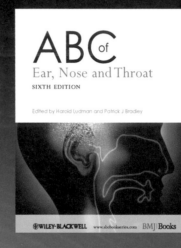
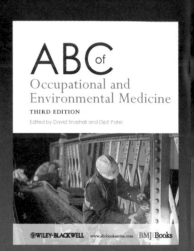
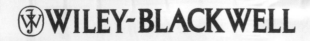

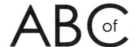

ABC of

Resuscitation

Sixth Edition

EDITORS

Jasmeet Soar FRCA FFICM FERC
Immediate Past Chair, Resuscitation Council (UK)
Consultant in Anaesthesia and Intensive Care Medicine
Southmead Hospital
North Bristol NHS Trust
Bristol, UK

Gavin D. Perkins MD FRCP FFICM FERC
Chair Advanced Life Support Subcommittee, Resuscitation Council (UK)
Clinical Professor of Critical Care Medicine
Warwick Medical School
University of Warwick
Coventry, UK

Jerry Nolan FRCA FRCP FCEM FFICM
Past Chair, Resuscitation Council (UK)
Consultant in Anaesthesia and Intensive Care Medicine
Royal United Hospital
Bath, UK

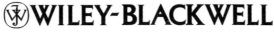

WILEY-BLACKWELL
A John Wiley & Sons, Ltd., Publication

BMJ|Books

Library of Congress Cataloging-in-Publication Data
ABC of resuscitation. –6th ed. / [edited by] Jasmeet Soar, Gavin D. Perkins, Jerry Nolan.
    p. ; cm. –(ABC series)
    Includes bibliographical references and index.
    Summary: "This book is a practical guide to the latest resuscitation advice for the non-specialist, and covers the core knowledge on the management of patients with cardiopulmonary arrest"–Provided by publisher.
    ISBN 978-0-470-67259-4 (pbk.)
    I. Soar, Jasmeet. II. Perkins, Gavin D. III. Nolan, Jerry. IV. Series: ABC series (Malden, Mass.)
    [DNLM: 1. Cardiopulmonary Resuscitation. WA 292]

    616.1–dc23

                                                                                              2012027833

A catalogue record for this book is available from the British Library.

Wiley also publishes its books in a variety of electronic formats. Some content that appears in print may not be available in electronic books.

Cover image: Cover photograph reproduced with kind permission by Michael Scott and the Resuscitation Council (UK).
Cover design by: Meaden Creative

Set in 9.25/12 Minion by Laserwords Private Limited, Chennai, India
Printed and bound in Malaysia by Vivar Printing Sdn Bhd

1   2013

Contents

List of Contributors

Sean Ainsworth, MBChB, FRCP(Edin), FRCPCH, DCH, MD

Consultant Paediatrician & Neonatologist, Neonatal Unit, Victoria Hospital, Kirkcaldy, UK

Robert Bingham, MB, BS, FRCA

Consultant Anaesthetist, Department of Anaesthesia, Great Ormond Street Children's Hospital, London, UK

Chair Paediatric Subcommittee, Resuscitation Council (UK)

Michael Colquhoun, BSc, MB, FRCP, MRCGP

Retired General Practitioner, Malvern, Worcestershire, UK

Chair, Basic Life Support Subcommittee, Resuscitation Council (UK)

Serena Cottrell, FRCPCH, MRCPI, BSc (Hons), MBBS, MMedSci

Consultant in Paediatric Emergency Medicine, Queen Alexandra Hospital, Portsmouth, UK

Lead for South Central Strategic Health Authority Child and Young Person's Advance Care Planning Working Group

Member of Executive Committee, Resuscitation Council (UK)

Keith Couper

Research Nurse, Heart of England NHS Foundation Trust, Birmingham, UK

Kate Crewdson, MB, BS, BSc

Specialist Registrar, Anaethesia and Intensive Care, Department of Anaesthesia, Bristol Royal Infirmary, Bristol, UK

Robin P. Davies RN

Resuscitation Council (UK) BLS/AED and ALS Subcommittee, Senior Resuscitation Officer, Heart of England NHS Foundation Trust, Birmingham, UK

Charles Deakin, MA, MD, FRCP, FRCA, FERC, FFICM

Consultant in Cardiac Anaesthesia and Intensive Care Medicine, University Hospital Southampton, Southampton, UK

Peter-Marc Fortune, BM, BSc, MA, PhD, FRCPCH, FFICM

Clinical Director of Critical Care, Royal Manchester Children's Hospital, Manchester, UK

Chair, Human Factors Working Group, Advanced Life Support Group, Salford, UK

David A. Gabbott, BM, BCh, MA, FRCA

Consultant Anaesthetist, Gloucestershire Hospitals NHS Foundation Trust, Department of Anaesthetics, Gloucester Royal Hospital, Gloucester, UK

Honorary Treasurer, Resuscitation Council (UK)

Carl Gwinnutt, MB, FRCA

Formerly Consultant Anaesthetist, Salford Royal Hospital NHS Foundation Trust, Salford, UK

Anthony J. Handley, MD, FRCP

Honorary Consultant Physician, Colchester Hospital University NHS Foundation Trust, Colchester, Essex, UK

Past Chair BLS/AED Subcommittee, Resuscitation Council (UK)

Andrew S. Lockey, MB ChB, MMedEd, FCEM, FIMC, FERC

Consultant in Emergency Medicine, Calderdale & Huddersfield NHS Foundation Trust, Accident and & Emergency Department, Calderdale Royal Hospital, Halifax, UK

Honorary Secretary, Resuscitation Council (UK)

David J. Lockey, MBBS, FRCA, FIMC, RCS(Ed), FACM

Consultant in Anaesthesia and Intensive Care, North Bristol NHS Trust

Honorary Professor, School of Clinical Sciences, University of Bristol, Bristol, UK

Ian K. Maconochie, FRCPCH, FCEM, FRCPI, FERC, PhD

Consultant in Paediatric Emergency Medicine, Paediatric Emergency Department, St Mary's Hospital, London, UK

Fionna P. Moore, MB, BS, BSc, FRCS, FRCSEd, FCEM, FIMC, RSCEd

Medical Director, London Ambulance Service NHS Trust, London, UK

Consultant in Emergency Medicine, Imperial College Healthcare Trust, London, UK

Jerry Nolan, FRCA, FRCP, FCEM, FFICM

Consultant in Anaesthesia and Intensive Care Medicine, Royal United Hospital, Bath, UK

Past Chair, Resuscitation Council (UK)

Gavin D. Perkins, MD, FRCP, FFICM, FERC

Professor of Critical Care Medicine, Warwick Medical School, University of Warwick, Coventry, UK

Consultant Physician, Heart of England NHS Foundation Trust, Birmingham, UK

Chair Advanced Life Support Subcommittee, Resuscitation Council (UK)

David Pitcher, MD, FRCP

Consultant Cardiologist, University Hospital, Birmingham, UK

Chair, Resuscitation Council (UK)

Susanna Price, MRCP, EDICM, FFICM, FESC

Consultant Cardiologist & Intensivist, Royal Brompton Hospital, London, UK

Rani Robson, BM, BCh, BSc (hons), MED, MRCP

Cardiology Registrar, Bristol Heart Institute, Bristol, UK

Gary B. Smith, BM Cert, MedEd, FHEA, FRCA, FRCP

Visiting Professor, Centre of Postgraduate Medical Research & Education (CoPMRE), The School of Health and Social Care, Bournemouth University, Bournemouth, UK

Joanne K. Smith, MSc (Cardiology)

Clinical Advisor to the Medical Directorate, London Ambulance Service NHS Trust, London, UK

Jasmeet Soar, FRCA, FFICM, FERC

Consultant in Anaesthesia and Intensive Care Medicine, Southmead Hospital, North Bristol NHS Trust, Bristol, UK

Immediate Past Chairman, Resuscitation Council (UK)

Mark Whitbread, MSc (Cardiology)

Consultant Paramedic, London Ambulance Service NHS Trust, London, UK

Jonathan Wyllie, MBChB, BSc, FRCP, FRCPCH, FERC

Consultant Neonatologist and Clinical Director of Neonatology, The James Cook University Hospital, Middlesbrough, UK Chair NLS Subcommittee, Resuscitation Council (UK)

Foreword

The birth of modern emergency first aid for cardiac arrest can be dated to the recognition that the newly described effective artificial ventilation together with chest compressions were 'parts of a whole and complete approach to resuscitation'. This occurred at a celebrated meeting of the pioneers of these techniques in 1960. By then, external defibrillators were also available. All that was needed was widespread dissemination of the necessary skills to permit the successful treatment of cardiac arrest to become an everyday reality. An international meeting to that end was held during the following year in Stavanger. At that time, chest compression was to be practised only by 'medical personnel, nurses, and recognised life savers'. Progress thereafter was inevitably slow. Guidelines for public use were first published in the USA in 1974, whilst in the UK a stimulus for healthcare professionals was provided by a series of articles published in the *British Medical Journal* during 1986 under the banner of 'The ABC of Resuscitation'. These were put together for the first edition of the booklet under that very apt name published at the end of the same year. The appearance now of a sixth edition attests its importance. It is based on the 2010 Guidelines of the Resuscitation Council (UK), has been prepared by the experts responsible for them and is greatly to be welcomed.

The booklet is not intended for the general public but rather for junior doctors, medical students, general practitioners, nurses and other healthcare professionals. There will be few healthcare professionals even with a major interest in resuscitation who will not benefit from its broad scope and the strong emphasis on key points. These are presented succinctly with commendable clarity that is aided by helpful illustrations. The 22 chapters include epidemiology, prevention, aetiology, clinical presentations, immediate managements, aftercare, devices, quality and ethics, all covering many situations through different ages from the newborn to adults.

Although all healthcare professionals do now receive training in resuscitation – and generally feel committed to good quality care – the skills are not easy to master. This is most true of chest compression which is performed to an excellent standard only rarely, as examination of tracings from real-time transmission or subsequent electronic downloads can attest. But it is not only compressions that are performed inadequately. All aspects of the prevention, management and aftercare of cardiac arrest suffer because they are practised infrequently, often in difficult environments, inevitably accompanied by anxiety and sometimes hindered by lack of confidence in the would-be rescuers. Constant revision of the principles and the details are needed if care is to be of a truly acceptable quality. No one strategy suffices to counter these difficulties but revision training, feedback and the ability readily to browse over the basics are all of paramount importance. The *ABC of Resuscitation* offers an excellent resource for the last of these requirements – as well as for initial training – to be valued by all who use it, and that will certainly include the writer of this Foreword.

Douglas Chamberlain
June 2012

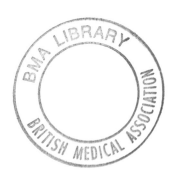

CHAPTER 1

Cardiac Arrest and the Chain of Survival

Jasmeet Soar[1], Gavin D. Perkins[2] and Jerry Nolan[3]

[1]Southmead Hospital, North Bristol NHS Trust, Bristol, UK
[2]Warwick Medical School, University of Warwick, Coventry, UK
[3]Royal United Hospital, Bath, UK

OVERVIEW

- Cardiovascular disease is the commonest cause of cardiac arrest
- Early recognition of warning signs and a call for help can prevent cardiac arrest
- If cardiac arrest occurs, immediate cardiopulmonary resuscitation (CPR) improves chances of survival
- Shockable cardiac arrest rhythms (ventricular fibrillation/pulseless ventricular tachycardia, VF/VT) are treated with attempted defibrillation
- Non-shockable rhythms (asystole and pulseless electrical activity (PEA)) are treated by identifying and treating the underlying cause.
- Post-cardiac arrest care in successfully resuscitated patients determines the final outcome

Epidemiology of cardiac arrest

In 2006, coronary heart disease accounted for 1 of every 6 deaths (a total of 425,425) in the United States and one-third of these deaths occurred within 1 h of symptom onset. In Europe, the annual incidence of emergency medical system (EMS)-treated, out-of-hospital cardiopulmonary arrest (OHCAs) for all rhythms is 40 per 100,000 population, with ventricular fibrillation (VF) arrest accounting for about one-third of these. However, data from recent studies indicate that the incidence of VF is declining: it was reported most recently as 23.7% among EMS-treated arrests of cardiac cause. Survival to hospital discharge is 8–10% for all-rhythm and around 21–27% for VF cardiac arrest; however, there is considerable regional variation in outcome.

The incidence of in-hospital cardiac arrest (IHCA) is difficult to assess because it is influenced heavily by factors such as the criteria for hospital admission and implementation of a Do Not Attempt Resuscitation (DNAR) policy. There are an estimated 200,000 treated IHCAs each year in the United States – approximately one per 1000 bed days. Of these patients undergoing CPR, 17.6% survive to hospital discharge and 13.6% have a favourable neurological outcome (Cerebral Performance Category (CPC) 1 or 2).

Many patients sustaining an IHCA have significant comorbidity, which influences the initial rhythm and, in these cases, strategies to prevent cardiac arrest are particularly important.

The chain of survival

The key steps for improving survival are shown in the chain of survival (Figure 1.1).

Early recognition and call for help

Out-of-hospital, early recognition of the importance of chest pain will enable the victim or a bystander to call the EMS and the victim to receive treatment that may prevent cardiac arrest. In-hospital, early recognition of the deteriorating patient who is at risk of cardiac arrest and a call for the resuscitation team or medical emergency team (MET) will enable treatment to prevent cardiac arrest. If cardiac arrest occurs, early recognition and a call for help are essential. Agonal breathing (gasping) often occurs immediately after cardiac arrest and is often mistaken for a sign of life – this can cause delays in starting CPR.

Early CPR

If cardiac arrest occurs, the victim will be unconscious, unresponsive and not breathing or not breathing normally (agonal breathing). Cardiopulmonary resuscitation (CPR) with chest compressions and ventilation of the victim's lungs will slow the deterioration of the brain and heart. Bystander CPR doubles the chances of long-term survival. Interruptions to chest compressions must be minimised

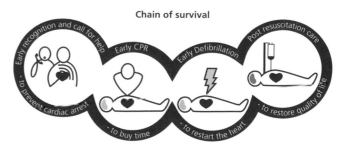

Chain of survival

Figure 1.1 Chain of survival.

ABC of Resuscitation, Sixth Edition. Edited by Jasmeet Soar, Gavin D. Perkins and Jerry Nolan.

and should occur only briefly during defibrillation attempts and rhythm checks.

Early defibrillation

Ventricular fibrillation (VF) is the commonest initial rhythm after a primary cardiac arrest although this often deteriorates to a non-shockable rhythm by the time it is first monitored. Early defibrillation can be effective at restoring a circulation. Public Access Defibrillation (PAD) programs using automated external defibrillators (AEDs) enable a wide range of rescuers to treat OHCA caused by VF. Most IHCAs tend to have an initial rhythm of pulseless electrical activity (PEA) or asystole but most survivors are among those with VF arrest. Hospital staff should therefore be trained and authorised to use a defibrillator (AED or manual) to enable the first responder to a cardiac arrest to attempt defibrillation when indicated, without delay.

Post resuscitation care

Return of a spontaneous circulation (ROSC) is an important phase in the continuum of resuscitation; however, the ultimate goal is a patient with normal cerebral function, a stable cardiac rhythm and normal haemodynamic function, so that they can leave hospital in good health and at minimum risk of a further cardiac arrest. The quality of the treatment given in the post-cardiac arrest phase will influence outcome – there is considerable inter-hospital variation in outcome among patients admitted to an intensive care unit after cardiac arrest (Box 1.1).

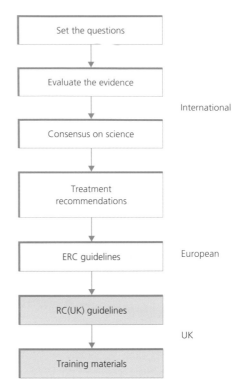

Figure 1.2 Resuscitation guidelines development process.

Consensus on Science and Treatment Recommendations (CoSTR). ILCOR (www.ilcor.org) therefore establishes the scientific evidence for the guidance and creates treatment recommendations (Figure 1.2).

Box 1.1 **Cardiac arrest statistics for the UK**

- Over 50,000 out-of-hospital cardiac arrests attended by the ambulance service
- About one-third of cardiac arrest victims have bystander CPR before an ambulance crew arrives
- About 30,000 in-hospital cardiac arrests each year
- Survival to discharge for out-of-hospital cardiac arrests is <10%
- Survival to discharge for in-hospital cardiac arrests is 10–20%

Resuscitation guidelines

The Resuscitation Council (UK) (www.resus.org.uk) provides healthcare professionals and laypeople with evidence-based guidelines for all patient groups (adults, children, newborn) and all settings. The scientific evidence supporting these guidelines is reviewed every 5 years (most recently in 2010). The UK Guidelines are based on the European Resuscitation Council (www.erc.edu) Guidelines. The European Guidelines are in turn derived from the International Liaison Committee on Resuscitation (ILCOR)

Further reading

Meaney PA, Nadkarni VM, Kern KB, *et al*. Rhythms and outcomes of adult in-hospital cardiac arrest. *Crit Care Med* 2010;**38**:101–8.

Merchant RM, Yang L, Becker LB, *et al*. Incidence of treated cardiac arrest in hospitalized patients in the United States. *Crit Care Med* 2011;**39**:2401–6.

Nichol G, Thomas E, Callaway CW, *et al*. Regional variation in out-of-hospital cardiac arrest incidence and outcome. *JAMA* 2008;**300**:1423–31.

Nolan JP, Soar J, Zideman DA, *et al*. on behalf of the ERC Guidelines Writing Group. European Resuscitation Council Guidelines for Resuscitation 2010: Section 1. Executive summary. *Resuscitation* 2010;**81**:219–76.

Nolan JP, Hazinski MF, Billi JE, *et al*. Part 1: Executive summary: 2010 International Consensus on Cardiopulmonary Resuscitation and Emergency Cardiovascular Care Science With Treatment Recommendations. *Resuscitation* 2010 Oct;**81**(Suppl 1):e1–25.

Nolan J, Soar J, Eikeland H. The chain of survival. *Resuscitation* 2006;**71**:270–1.

Resuscitation Council (UK). Resuscitation Guidelines 2010. Available at http://www.resus.org.uk/pages/guide.htm.

Sasson C, Rogers MA, Dahl J, Kellermann AL. Predictors of survival from out-of-hospital cardiac arrest: a systematic review and meta-analysis. *Circ Cardiovasc Qual Outcomes* 2010;**3**:63–81.

CHAPTER 2

Sudden Cardiac Death

David Pitcher

University Hospital Birmingham, UK

OVERVIEW

- SCD can occur at any age, but its frequency increases with increasing age and its causes vary with age
- Ischaemic heart disease is the commonest cause of SCD in people older than 35 years
- Inherited conditions are more common in people below the age of 35
- Warning signs are often absent, but can include chest pain, shortness of breath and syncope
- Identification and treatment of the underlying condition under specialist guidance can prevent SCD

Introduction

Sudden cardiac death (SCD) is defined as 'Natural death due to cardiac causes, heralded by abrupt loss of consciousness within 1 hour of the onset of acute symptoms; pre-existing heart disease may have been known to have been present but the time and mode of death are unexpected'. In this chapter we shall consider causes of sudden cardiac death in adults, how to identify those at potential risk of sudden death, and what treatment options may prevent or reduce the risk of sudden death.

Causes of sudden cardiac death

Sudden cardiac death may occur at any age, but its frequency increases with age and its causes vary with age. Causes may be inherited or acquired (or a combination of both). Coronary atheroma and resulting ischaemic heart disease are the commonest cause of SCD in adults over the age of 35 but other, predominantly acquired, conditions can cause SCD in this age group. Inherited conditions are a less common cause in older adults but predominate as the cause of SCD in people below the age of 35. Table 2.1 lists some of the important causes.

ABC of Resuscitation, Sixth Edition. Edited by Jasmeet Soar, Gavin D. Perkins and Jerry Nolan.

How do people present?

Sadly, many people present by dying suddenly; the first doctor to assess them is the coroner's pathologist. The autopsy is really important in this tragic situation, because it may provide information that will allow prevention of SCD in other family members. Some inherited conditions that predispose to SCD, such as hypertrophic cardiomyopathy (HCM) and arrhythmogenic right ventricular cardiomyopathy (ARVC), may not be easy to confirm or exclude at a routine autopsy and detailed examination of hearts of SCD victims by an expert cardiac pathologist is recommended. When an autopsy identifies an inherited abnormality, there is an opportunity to screen family members to identify others at risk, in whom treatment may prevent SCD. When autopsy finds no abnormality to explain death, this is regarded as sudden adult death syndrome (SADS). This should always trigger consideration of whether or not there may have been a purely 'electrical' inherited cardiac condition that may be present in other family members.

Some people present with 'failed sudden death', when a person suffers cardiac arrest from which cardiopulmonary resuscitation (CPR) is successful. Increased public access to effective CPR and early defibrillation has increased the incidence of this situation. This provides an important opportunity to assess and offer preventative treatment to the survivor of the arrest and, when there is an inherited cause, to family members at risk. Healthcare professionals involved in successful resuscitation from cardiac arrest and in post-resuscitation care have a unique opportunity to identify individuals with a high risk of further cardiac arrest and those who have an inherited basis for cardiac arrest, with implications for family members.

Some people at risk of SCD experience warning symptoms. In people with severe coronary disease the warning symptom is likely to be angina or an acute coronary syndrome. In people with severe aortic stenosis it may be angina, breathlessness or syncope. People at risk of sudden death from cardiac arrhythmia may experience syncope. When someone presents after syncope, they should be assessed to identify features of common problems that do not carry a significant risk of death (such as uncomplicated faints) and to identify a small minority in whom syncope is the only prior warning of a life-threatening but treatable problem. This problem might be, for example, high-grade atrioventricular

Table 2.1 Some causes of sudden cardiac death.

Condition	Causes	Further detail
Long QT syndromes (LQTS)	Inherited (autosomal dominant) ion channel disorders Many different genotypes but types 1–3 are most common	Predispose to *torsade de pointes* VT and VF
Acquired QT interval prolongation	Drug therapy Ischaemic heart disease Myocarditis	Predisposes to *torsade de pointes* VT and VF
Brugada syndrome	Inherited (autosomal dominant) ion channel disorder	Occurs worldwide but more common in SE Asia. Risk of SCD higher in young males
Short QT syndrome (SQTS)	Rare, inherited (autosomal dominant) ion channel disorder	Predisposes to *torsade de pointes* VT and VF
Catecholaminergic polymorphic ventricular tachycardia (CPVT)	Rare, inherited (autosomal dominant) ion channel disorder	Predisposes to *torsade de pointes* VT and VF, especially on exercise
Arrhythmogenic right ventricular cardiomyopathy (ARVC)	Inherited (autosomal dominant)	Predisposes to VT and VF
Hypertrophic cardiomyopathy (HCM)	Inherited (autosomal dominant) Several different genotypes	SCD risk is due to VT and VF. Risk varies with genotype and with individual factors
Wolff–Parkinson–White (WPW) syndrome	Mostly sporadic Infrequent familial incidence	Not all WPW patients are at risk of SCD. Risk is due to rapid transmission of AF to the ventricles, triggering VT or VF
High-grade atrioventricular block	Conducting system fibrosis Calcific aortic stenosis Myocardial diseases including ischaemic heart disease Cardiac surgery Drug therapy Occasionally congenital	Predisposes to ventricular standstill (asystole). Some people with extreme bradycardia develop *torsade de pointes* VT and VF
Severe aortic stenosis	Congenital bicuspid valve (becomes severe at age 50–70 or younger) Degenerative (becomes severe in elderly patients)	If untreated may progress to heart failure or SCD, probably mostly due to VT or VF
Dilated cardiomyopathy	Probably multiple causes Familial in a minority of cases	Many develop progressive heart failure but there is risk of SCD due to VT or VF
Ischaemic heart disease due to coronary atheroma	Partly genetic, partly acquired	SCD risk is mainly due to VT or VF, which may be in response to acute ischaemia or infarction or may be due to previous myocardial scarring
Other myocardial diseases	Hypertensive heart disease, sarcoid heart disease, etc.	May predispose to ventricular arrhythmia or AVB in some patients
Anomalous coronary artery anatomy	Congenital	Rare cause of SCD in young people, often on exercise. Risk varies with the anomalous anatomical pattern

SCD = sudden cardiac death; VT = ventricular tachycardia; VF = ventricular fibrillation; AF = atrial fibrillation.

block (AVB), as shown in Figure 2.1, in which a pacemaker will protect against SCD, or an inherited cardiac condition predisposing to ventricular arrhythmia, requiring an implanted cardioverter-defibrillator (ICD) in some patients.

Other modes of presentation are by screening or by chance identification of a potential risk. In addition to screening relatives of SCD or cardiac arrest victims, there is an increasing focus on screening participants in competitive sport to try to prevent sudden death on the sports field, and some people are found to have clinical evidence of structural heart disease or an ECG abnormality when being assessed for other reasons.

Inherited cardiac conditions

Although relatively uncommon as a cause of SCD, it is important that those providing CPR are aware of inherited cardiac conditions and are able to recognise those who may have them. They cause SCD by predisposing to sudden ventricular arrhythmia: ventricular tachycardia (VT), including *torsade de pointes* (Figure 2.2), and ventricular fibrillation (VF). Ion channel disorders such as long QT syndromes (LQTS), Brugada syndrome, catecholaminergic poly-morphic ventricular tachycardia (CPVT) and short QT syndrome occur without any structural heart disease; some of these can be

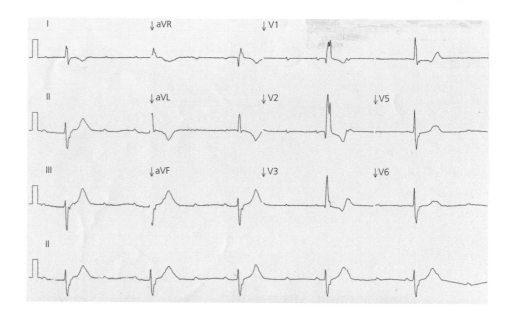

Figure 2.1 ECG showing broad-complex complete atrioventricular block.

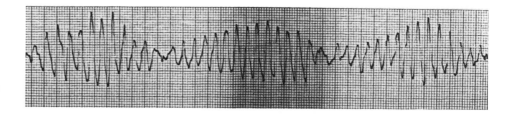

Figure 2.2 ECG showing *torsade de pointes* ventricular tachycardia.

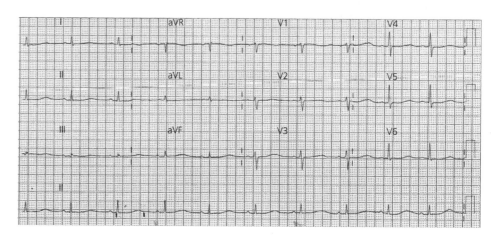

Figure 2.3 ECG showing prolonged QT interval in a patient with long QT syndrome.

identified from typical ECG features. An example of an ECG in LQTS is shown in Figure 2.3 and a typical Brugada syndrome ECG is shown in Figure 2.4. Some people with these conditions may have a normal resting ECG and diagnosis may require provocative testing, such as exercise testing or catecholamine challenge for CPVT or flecainide or ajmaline testing for Brugada syndrome.

Other inherited conditions involve abnormalities of cardiac structure and function. These include HCM and ARVC, and a minority of cases of dilated cardiomyopathy (DCM) also has a familial basis.

Consideration of genetic testing is appropriate when an inherited cardiac condition is identified in an individual. Patients who have been resuscitated from unexplained cardiac arrest or who have unexplained syncope should undergo specialist assessment in a unit with expertise in detecting and treating inherited cardiac conditions.

Prevention of sudden cardiac death

In some people, reducing risk of SCD requires avoidance of specific activities or circumstances that predispose to SCD.

In some this will mean abstaining from vigorous exercise. In most parts of the world, HCM is the commonest cause of SCD during sport (Figure 2.5). The exception is Italy, where pre-participation screening has been performed for many years, and people with HCM have not been permitted to engage in

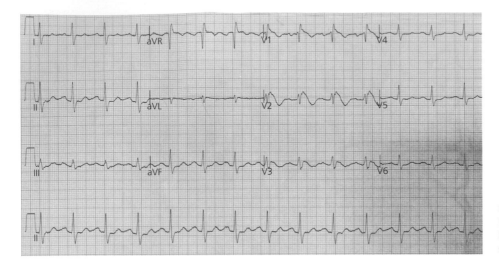

Figure 2.4 ECG showing typical features of Brugada syndrome. Note the right bundle branch block morphology and unusual ST segment elevation in leads V1-V3.

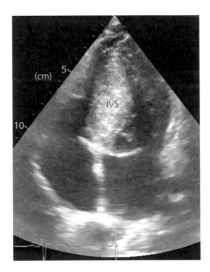

Figure 2.5 Echocardiogram showing an apical 4-chamber view from a patient with hypertrophic cardiomyopathy. He presented after a syncopal attack whilst running, was found to have features indicating a high risk of SCD, advised to refrain from vigorous exercise and to undergo ICD implantation. Note the very thick interventricular septum (normal up to 1.2 cm). IVS, interventricular septum; LA, left atrium; LV, left ventricle; RA, right atrium; RV, right ventricle.

competitive sport. Although there is an ongoing debate regarding the optimal screening methods, increasing screening of sportspeople offers an opportunity to identify and protect those at highest risk; this will include those with other inherited cardiac conditions as well as HCM. When the ECG is used for screening, it should be interpreted by someone with expertise in distinguishing true abnormalities from features that represent physiological adaptation to high-level exercise training.

People with LQTS should avoid drugs that cause further QT prolongation (including amiodarone, which in a resuscitation setting would otherwise be used to treat VT) and avoid hypokalaemia (e.g. due to thiazide-like diuretics). The circumstances in which SCD occurs varies, depending on the underlying condition and by no means all are related to exercise. For example, in LQTS type 2, SCD may be triggered by a sudden noise (e.g. an alarm clock or fire

alarm), whereas in LQTS type 3 and Brugada syndrome, SCD is more likely at rest, such as during sleep. Alterations of lifestyle or activity to reduce risk should be tailored to the specific condition in each individual.

Specific treatment will reduce risk of SCD in many of the situations outlined here.

Coronary atheroma and ischaemic heart disease

Detailed discussion of measures that may reduce progression of and risk of SCD from this condition is beyond the scope of this chapter. It is important to identify those at high risk of premature or severe coronary disease, such as those with familial dyslipidaemia, since early, effective treatment may prevent or delay development of severe, life-threatening coronary disease. In those with symptoms from coronary disease, prompt assessment and appropriate treatment can reduce the risk of SCD. This applies especially in those with acute ST-segment-elevation myocardial infarction in whom immediate reperfusion therapy and appropriate drug therapy will reduce the risk of future SCD, by minimising myocardial damage and resulting left ventricular impairment. The latest European guidance on both prevention and treatment of coronary disease can be accessed at www.escardio.org.

Heart failure and left ventricular systolic impairment

Detailed consideration of the treatment of heart failure is beyond the scope of this chapter. People who have experienced heart failure or who have substantial impairment of left ventricular systolic function are at increased risk of SCD; that risk can be minimised by appropriate treatment. For many that will involve optimal medical treatment, but for selected patients the use of an implanted device to provide cardiac resynchronisation therapy (biventricular pacing), with or without an ICD capability, will reduce further the risk of SCD. Patients with heart failure require risk assessment to determine the most appropriate treatment for each individual. The latest European guidance on treatment of heart failure can be accessed at www.escardio.org.

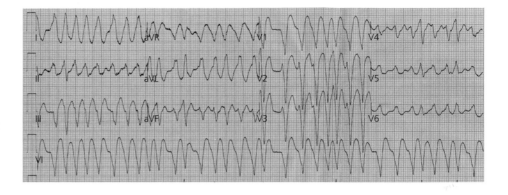

Figure 2.6 ECG showing pre-excited atrial fibrillation in a patient with Wolff–Parkinson–White syndrome. Note that the rhythm is irregular and the rate fast. The QRS complexes are broad, with a slurred upstroke, and their morphology varies from beat to beat.

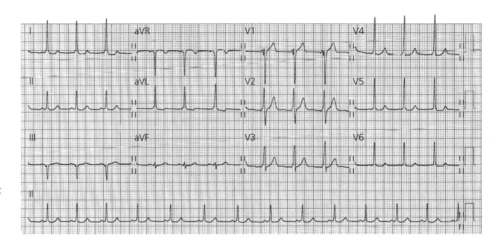

Figure 2.7 ECG showing typical ventricular pre-excitation during sinus rhythm in a patient with Wolff–Parkinson–White syndrome. The short PR interval and delta wave are seen best in leads I, and V1–V4.

Long QT syndromes

In people with LQTS (especially types 1 and 2), treatment with a beta-adrenoceptor blocking drug will reduce SCD risk to a very low level. In some of these patients, SCD risk may also be reduced by pacemaker implantation.

Severe aortic stenosis

In people with severe aortic stenosis, the risk of SCD is reduced by valve replacement.

Atrio-ventricular block

In people with high-grade atrio-ventricular block (AVB), pacemaker implantation reduces the risk of SCD, so should be considered even in the absence of symptoms. Other causes of bradycardia (e.g. sinus node disease) are not associated with a high risk of SCD and the need for pacing is dictated by symptoms.

Wolff–Parkinson–White syndrome

Although a rare cause of SCD, this syndrome deserves mention. Some, but not all, patients with ventricular pre-excitation have an increased risk of SCD. This is believed to occur when atrial fibrillation (AF) develops and is transmitted rapidly to the ventricles via the accessory pathway, triggering VT and VF. People who present with pre-excited AF (Figure 2.6) with rapid heart rates are likely to be at risk in this way. Others with pre-excitation on

their ECG in sinus rhythm (Figure 2.7) require risk assessment by electrophysiology studies. Radiofrequency ablation of the accessory pathway will prevent SCD due to AF in those at risk.

However, in some of these clinical settings there is either no such specific treatment to reduce risk, or there is substantial residual risk despite appropriate treatment. In these people, implantation of an ICD to provide prompt termination of potentially fatal ventricular arrhythmia should be considered. This may be in the context of 'secondary prevention' in a person who has already had a life-threatening event, or as 'primary prevention' in people identified to have a high risk of SCD that cannot be reduced adequately by other treatment. Implantation of an ICD carries some risk and has other implications on lifestyle, as well as some psychological impact. In any person who has been resuscitated from cardiac arrest, or who has been identified as being at risk of SCD that is not correctable using other treatment, the relative risks and benefits of ICD implantation should be considered by a cardiologist with expertise in assessment and treatment of heart rhythm disorders.

Further reading

Basso C, Burke M, Fornes P, *et al.* Guidelines for autopsy investigation of sudden cardiac death. *Virchows Arch* 2008;**452**(1):11–8.

Corrado D, Pellicia A, Heidbuchel H, *et al.* Recommendations for interpretation of 12-lead electrocardiogram in the athlete. *Eur Heart J* 2010;**31**:243–59.

Dickstein K, Vardas PE, Auricchio A, *et al.* 2010 Focused Update of ESC Guidelines on device therapy in heart failure. *Eur Heart J* 2010;**31**:2677–87.

Drezner JA, Khan K. Sudden cardiac death in young athletes. Evidence supports a systematic screening programme before participation. *BMJ* 2008;**337**:61–2.

Elliott P, McKenna WJ. Hypertrophic cardiomyopathy. *Lancet* 2004;**363**: 1881–91.

Maron BJ, Zipes DP. 36th Bethesda Conference: Eligibility Recommendations for Competitive Athletes with Cardiovascular Abnormalities. *J Am Coll Cardiol* 2005;**45**:1313–75.

Morita H, Wu J, Zipes D. The QT syndromes: long and short. *Lancet* 2008;**372**:750–63.

National Institute for Health and Clinical Excellence. Implantable cardioverter defibrillators for arrhythmias. Review of Technology Appraisal 11. 2006. http://www.nice.org.uk/nicemedia/live/11566/33167/33167.pdf.

National Institute for Health and Clinical Excellence. Management of transient loss of consciousness in adults and young people. 2010. http://www.nice.org.uk/nicemedia/live/13111/50452/50452.pdf.

Northcote RJ, Ballantyne D. Sudden cardiac death in sport. *BMJ* 1983;**287**: 1357–59.

Zipes DP, Camm AJ, Borggrefe M, *et al*. ACC/AHA/ESC 2006 guidelines for management of patients with ventricular arrhythmias and the prevention of sudden cardiac death. *Eur Heart J* 2006;**8**:746–837.

CHAPTER 3

Causes and Prevention of Cardiac Arrest in Hospital

Gary B. Smith

The School of Health and Social Care, Bournemouth University, Bournemouth, UK

OVERVIEW

- Overall survival to hospital discharge following in-hospital cardiac arrest (IHCA) in adults is < 20%
- Most IHCAs occur during non-cardiac illness and are heralded by unrecognised, or untreated, slow and progressive respiratory and circulatory deterioration due to the patent's underlying admission diagnosis, associated complications or coexisting diseases
- False cardiac arrests often signify unrecognised pathology and have a high subsequent in-hospital mortality (20–30%)
- Hospitals can structure their processes for the prevention of patient deterioration and cardiac arrest using the 'chain of prevention' – a five-ringed chain comprising education, monitoring, recognition, call for help and response
- There are considerable opportunities for reducing the incidence of IHCA by better use of 'do not attempt cardiopulmonary resuscitation' (DNACPR) decisions and end-of-life (EoL) care in patients where the underlying condition and patient's general health makes the success of cardiopulmonary resuscitation (CPR) unlikely

---

Introduction

Most in-hospital cardiac arrests (IHCAs) are predictable events associated with slow and progressive deterioration in the patient's cardiac, respiratory and neurological function due to a non-cardiac problem. Overall survival to hospital discharge following IHCA in adults is < 20%. Therefore, measures aimed at preventing IHCA are essential to improving outcome for at-risk patients.

Demographics of IHCA

The distribution of IHCA usually depends upon the hospital's proportion of intensive care unit (ICU) and high-dependency care unit (HDU) beds. These beds are usually equipped with continuous or automated patient vital signs monitoring. Hospitals with a high proportion of ICU and HDU beds tend to have a greater proportion

ABC of Resuscitation, Sixth Edition. Edited by Jasmeet Soar, Gavin D. Perkins and Jerry Nolan.
© 2013 John Wiley & Sons, Ltd. Published 2013 by John Wiley & Sons, Ltd.

of cardiac arrests occurring in monitored patients. In hospitals with few such beds, most arrests occur in unmonitored patients and are usually also unwitnessed. Irrespective of arrest location, the primary cardiac arrest rhythm in hospital is usually either asystole or pulseless electrical activity (PEA).

Outcome following in-hospital cardiac arrest

Only about 15–20% of patients suffering an IHCA survive to hospital discharge. Survival is better if the arrest occurs in a monitored area, is witnessed, or the victim has a shockable rhythm (i.e. ventricular fibrillation or pulseless ventricular tachycardia). Most adult survivors of IHCA are defibrillated immediately. Many IHCA survivors have a full return of neurological status to pre-arrest levels, but approximately 40% may have moderate or severe neurological disability. Although cardiac arrest is rare in hospitalised pregnant women and children, the underlying causes are similar and outcomes are similarly poor.

Predisposing factors

Hospitalised patients with an admission diagnosis of heart disease may suffer a cardiac arrest caused by a sudden change in cardiac rhythm due to an irritable myocardium. However, most IHCAs occur during non-cardiac illness and are heralded by unrecognised, or untreated, respiratory and circulatory deterioration due to the patent's underlying admission diagnosis, associated complications or coexisting diseases (e.g. hypertension, diabetes mellitus, renal disease).

IHCA is rare in pregnant women, but when it occurs it can often also be linked to a failure of prompt recognition of physiological deterioration by hospital staff. Specific risks that may predispose to deterioration include pre-existing medical conditions, maternal sepsis, eclampsia and obstetric haemorrhage. In children, cardiac arrest due to primary cardiac disease is extremely rare. More often profound hypoxaemia and hypotension are the cause, with asystole or PEA being the most common initial arrest rhythms.

The role of 'false' arrests

A 'false' arrest can be defined as an IHCA call for which no cardiopulmonary resuscitation (CPR) is needed. This usually occurs when one of the following exists: (a) a cardiac arrest call is cancelled by the hospital telephone exchange soon after having been made; (b) the patient is found to have been dead for some time and no CPR is undertaken by the resuscitation team; or (c) the patient is found not to have suffered a cardiac arrest. The false arrest is often caused by one of the conditions shown in Box 3.1. Particular attention should be paid to patients who have a 'false cardiac arrest', as the event often signifies unrecognised illness. The subsequent hospital mortality for patients suffering a false cardiac arrest is approximately 20–30%.

Box 3.1 Events associated with 'false' cardiac arrests calls in hospital

- Vasovagal collapse
- Chest pain
- Respiratory depression
- Morphine overdose
- Postoperative bleeding
- Tachycardia
- Bradycardia
- Hypoxia
- Sudden reduction in conscious level
- Seizures

Other factors influencing the occurrence of IHCA

Adequate patient monitoring and assessment are crucial to preventing adverse outcomes, such as IHCA. Ideally, the sickest patients should be admitted to areas that can provide the greatest supervision and the highest level of nursing care and organ support. Higher nurse–patient staffing ratios are associated with a reduction in IHCA rates. IHCA survival rates are lower during nights and weekends. Hospital processes, such as admission to hospital at night or at weekends, or discharge from an ICU to a general ward at night, also increase the risk of cardiac arrest and death.

Structuring systems to prevent patient deterioration and cardiac arrest in hospital

The essential components of a system for preventing patient deterioration and IHCA are described by the 'chain of prevention' and shown in Figure 3.1. Each component is represented by a ring in the chain. The rings are education, monitoring, recognition, call for help and response.

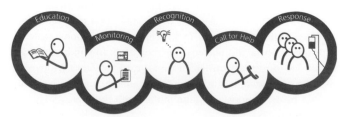

Figure 3.1 The chain of prevention (from Smith GB. In-hospital cardiac arrest: Is it time for an in-hospital 'chain of prevention'? Resuscitation 2010;81:1209–11.). Reproduced by permission of Professor Gary B. Smith. Copyright © 2012 Gary B. Smith.

As no chain is stronger than its weakest link, failure (or absence) of one or more of its components (rings) will inevitably result in failure of the whole system. This will be manifested by patient deterioration and cardiac arrest. If the components of the chain are present and strong, the chain will work perfectly, and this should be measureable as a reduction in the number of preventable IHCAs.

The first ring of the chain of prevention: staff education

Research suggests that some medical and nursing staff do not possess the knowledge, skills or confidence to deal with acutely ill patients in general hospital wards. Often there is a failure to use a systematic approach to the assessment of critically ill patients; poor communication; a lack of teamwork and insufficient use of treatment limitation plans. Evidence of reduced IHCA rates after educational interventions is emerging.

Hospitals need to ensure that their staff have the necessary competencies to recognise the signs of patient deterioration and to manage the acutely ill patient. The exact competencies required will vary between staff groups, but all members of clinical staff should be competent to undertake the activities shown in Box 3.2.

Box 3.2 Acute care competencies that all clinical staff should possess

- The ability to observe patients correctly and to measure and record patient's vital signs
- The knowledge to interpret observed findings
- The ability to recognise the signs of deterioration
- The ability to use an early warning scoring system or 'calling criteria'
- The ability to appreciate the level of clinical urgency required by a given situation
- The ability to use simple interventions (airway opening, oxygen therapy, intravenous fluid administration, etc)
- The ability to work successfully as part of a multiprofessional team
- The ability to organise care appropriately
- The knowledge of how to seek help from other staff
- The knowledge to use a systematic approach to information delivery, e.g. RSVP or SBAR
- The ability to initiate or facilitate discussions about 'do not attempt cardiopulmonary resuscitation' (DNACPR) decisions and end-of-life (EoL) care

---

The second ring of the chain of prevention: monitoring

Clinical deterioration is virtually always accompanied by abnormalities of breathing rate, pulse rate, temperature, blood pressure, conscious level or SpO_2, and by 'non-specific' signs such as pallor and diaphoresis. This relationship forms the basis for repeated clinical observation and monitoring of patients' vital signs in hospital. Despite this, numerous studies suggest that the frequent reassessment of clinical status does not always occur; vital signs datasets are also often found to be incomplete.

Improvements in clinical observation can be achieved by establishing a vital signs monitoring plan for each patient on admission that is based on the patient's age, admission diagnosis and co-morbidities, and which identifies the vital signs variables to be measured and the frequency of measurement. Suggested physiological parameters for routine measurement in patients admitted to hospital are shown in Box 3.3. The frequency and type of observations should be matched to the patient's severity of illness; monitoring regimens should alter each time a patient's condition changes. In future, the reliability of vital signs monitoring might be achieved using continuous monitoring technology, but existing systems are prone to generating false positive alarms.

Box 3.3 **Suggested physiological parameters for routine measurement in patients admitted to hospital**

- Heart rate (pulse rate)
- Breathing rate
- Blood pressure
- Temperature
- Conscious level (using AVPU [**A**lert–Responds to **V**oice–Responds to **P**ain–**U**nresponsive])
- S_pO_2
- Inspired oxygen

The third ring of the chain of prevention: recognition

Alterations in a patient's vital signs, singly or in combination, are associated with the occurrence of IHCA, hospital death and unplanned ICU admission with varying sensitivity and specificity. These patterns can be difficult to spot in a busy general ward. Consequently, many hospitals now use early warning scores (EWS)

or 'calling criteria' to assist in the early detection of critical illness. Both rely upon the regular monitoring of vital signs. EWS systems allocate weightings to routine vital sign measurements on the basis of their deviation from a pre-defined 'normal' range (Figures 3.2 and 3.3).

EWS or 'calling criteria' systems require the development of unambiguous, mandatory activation protocols for escalating monitoring or summoning a response to a deteriorating patient. Early warning scoring systems use the sum of all measurement weightings (the EWS) to determine the time to the next vital signs observation set or to mandate a call to a rapid response team (RRT) (Figure 3.4). Systems incorporating 'calling criteria' usually activate a RRT response when one or more routinely measured physiological variable reaches an extremely abnormal value (Figure 3.5). The EWS systems offer a graded escalation of care, whereas 'calling criteria' provide an all-or-nothing response. Whilst most hospitals find the use of EWS or 'calling criteria' systems useful, the sensitivity, specificity, and accuracy of these systems to identify patients at risk of IHCA have been poorly investigated to date.

Other recent developments that may improve the detection of patient deterioration include (a) better design of vital signs charts, (b) the use of sophisticated vital signs charting technology and (c) monitoring technology incorporating complex escalation algorithms.

The fourth ring of the chain of prevention: call for help

Failure of ward staff to call for assistance from more experienced personnel is a common finding in case reviews of patients who deteriorate. Failure occurs because few staff have been trained to pass on information about patient deterioration in a structured way, and because of worry on the part of the caller that their clinical judgement may be criticised if they do call for help. Communication

Score	3	2	1	0	1	2	3
Respiratory rate (bpm)	≤8		9–11	12–20		21–24	≥25
S_pO_2 (%)	≤91	92–93	94–95	≥96			
Any supplemental oxygen?		Yes		No			
Temperature (°C)	≤35.0		35.1–36.0	36.1–38.0	38.1–39.0	≥39.1	
Systolic BP (mm Hg)	≤90	91–100	101–110	111–219			≥220
Heart rate (bpm)	≤40		41–50	51–90	91–110	111–130	≥131
Conscious level (using AVPU system)				Alert (A)			Voice (V) Pain (P) Unresponsive (U)

Figure 3.2 An example of an Early Warning Score. This is the National Early Warning Score (NEWS). bpm, beats per minute; AVPU, **A**lert–Responds to **V**oice–Responds to **P**ain–**U**nresponsive. (Modified from Royal College of Physicians 2012.).

Score	3	2	1	0	1	2	3
Respiratory rate (bpm)	≤8		9–11	12–20		(21–24)	≥25
S$_p$O$_2$ (%)	≤91	92–93	(94–95)	≥96			
Any supplemental oxygen?		(Yes)		No			
Temperature (°C)	≤35.0		35.1–36.0	36.1–38.0	(38.1–39.0)	≥39.1	
Systolic BP (mm Hg)	≤90	(91–100)	101–110	111–219			≥220
Heart rate (bpm)	≤40		41–50	51–90	(91–110)	111–130	≥131
Conscious level (using AVPU system)				Alert (A)			(Voice (V) Pain (P) Unresponsive (U))

Figure 3.3 Calculation of an EWS using NEWS. This example illustrates the weighted values allocated to the following physiological measurements: respiratory rate = 22 breaths.min^{-1}; SpO2 = 95%; inspired gas = oxygen; temperature = 38.7 °C; systolic BP = 95 mmHg; pulse = 109 beats.min^{-1}; conscious level = responds to voice. The resultant NEWS value is $2 + 1 + 2 + 1 + 1 + 2 + 3 = 12$. bpm, beats per minute; AVPU, **A**lert–Responds to **V**oice–Responds to **P**ain–**U**nresponsive. (Modified from Royal College of Physicians 2012.).

RRT calling criteria	
Airway	Threatened
Breathing	All respiratory arrests Respiratory rate <5 Respiratory rate >30
Circulation	All cardiac arrests Pulse rate <40 Pulse rate >140
Neurology	Sudden fall in level of consciousness (e.g., fall in GCS of > 2 points) Repeated or prolonged seizures
Other	Any patient that you are seriously worried about that does not fit the above criteria

Figure 3.4 Typical Rapid Response Team calling criteria. GCS, Glasgow Coma Scale.

NEWS score	Minimum observation frequency	Clinical response
0	12 hourly	• Continue routine NEWS monitoring with every set of observations.
1 – 4	4 – 6 hourly	• Inform registered nurse who must assess the patient. • Registered nurse to decide if increased frequency of monitoring and/ or escalation of clinical care is required.
>5 or a score of 3 in any single parameter	1 hourly	• Registered nurse to urgently inform the medical team caring for the patient. • Urgent assessment by a clinician with core competencies to assess acutely ill patients. • Clinical care in an environment with monitoring facilities.
≥7	Continuous monitoring of vital signs	• Registered nurse to immediately inform the medical team caring for the patient–this should be at least at Specialist Registar level. • Emergency assessment by a clinical team with critical care competencies, which also includes a practitioner/s with advanced airway skills. • Consider transfer of clinical care to a level 2 or 3 care facility, i.e. high dependency or critical care unit.

Figure 3.5 Graded escalation criteria for National Early Warning Score (NEWS).

could be improved if hospitals ensured that all staff are empowered to call for help whenever they feel they need it and if structured communication tools, such as RSVP (Reason–Story–Vital Signs–Plan) or SBAR (Situation–Background–Assessment–Recommendation), are used to ensure effective inter-professional communication. In some hospitals, the patient's family and friends are also encouraged to call the RRT.

The fifth ring of the chain of prevention: response

Once the call for assistance for more experienced help has been made by ward staff, the response needs to be both appropriate and speedy. Although many publications report that responding staff often only employ simple tasks, such as starting oxygen therapy and/or intravenous fluids, an Australian study suggested that all nearly all calls to a RRT required 'critical care-type' interventions. However, not all responding staff possess the necessary critical care skills to stabilise deteriorating patients and their response may also often be slow. To counter this, many hospitals now use specifically created RRTs known as critical care outreach teams (CCOT) or medical emergency teams (MET). CCOTs are usually nurse-led, whilst other RRTs may be formed of medical and nursing staff from intensive care and general medicine. Both types respond to specific EWS values or 'calling criteria'. RRTs for paediatric and maternity services have also been described.

Evidence of an impact of RRTs on reducing IHCA rates is variable. Numerous single-centre studies have reported reduced numbers of IHCAs, but a cluster-randomised controlled trial of the MET system was unable to confirm an impact. A *post hoc* analysis of the same data showed that there was a decrease in IHCA with increased activation of the MET system. However, a recent meta-analysis showed that RRT systems were associated with a reduction in rates of cardiopulmonary arrest outside the ICU but not with lower hospital mortality rates.

The role of 'do not attempt cardiopulmonary resuscitation' decisions in reducing the cardiac arrest rate in hospital

Most people now die in hospital, where advanced CPR techniques can, in practice, be offered to any patient. However, all too often, CPR is started when the underlying condition and general health of the patient makes success unlikely. In these cases, there are considerable opportunities for reducing the incidence of IHCA requiring CPR if 'do not attempt cardiopulmonary resuscitation' (DNACPR) decision-making and end-of-life (EoL) care planning are considered early in the patient's admission.

Suggested guidelines for the prevention of in-hospital cardiac arrest

Box 3.4 describes suggested guidelines for the prevention of in-hospital cardiac arrest, using the principles of the 'chain of prevention'.

Box 3.4 **Guidelines for prevention of in-hospital cardiac arrest**

1 Locate patients in an area of the hospital where the level of care provided is matched to the patient's level of illness
2 Use the 'chain of prevention' as a basis for the structuring of responses to patient deterioration and the prevention of cardiopulmonary arrest
3 Train all clinical staff in the recognition, monitoring and management of the at-risk or critically ill patient. This training should include advice on the necessary clinical management required whilst awaiting the arrival of more experienced staff. Inform all staff of their role(s) in the rapid response system
4 Ensure that all patients have a documented, individualised vital signs monitoring and observation plan. The plan should identify which variables need to be measured and the frequency of measurement. Current opinion and research evidence suggests that the important variables are pulse, blood pressure, respiratory rate, conscious level, temperature, SpO_2 and inspired oxygen concentration (i.e. air/oxygen) at the time of SpO_2 measurement
5 Use a system to facilitate the early detection of patient deterioration (i.e. either an early warning scoring system or 'calling criteria') on a routine basis
6 Use a patient chart, or electronic vital signs charting system, that facilitates the regular measurement and recording of vital signs and, where used, early warning scores
7 Establish a clear, unambiguous, mandatory, graded, activation protocol for escalating monitoring or summoning a response to a deteriorating patient. This should include advice on the further clinical management of the patient and the specific responsibilities of medical and nursing staff
8 Empower staff of all disciplines, and perhaps also patients' relatives to call for help when they identify a patient at risk of deterioration or cardiac arrest, or are concerned about the patient's condition
9 Use a single structured communication tool (e.g. SBAR, RSVP) throughout the organisation to ensure effective handover of information between doctors, nurses and other healthcare professions. Ensure that all staff are trained to use the tool
10 Establish a clear and specific response to critical illness, over and above that provided by the patient's primary team. This may include a designated critical care outreach or medical emergency team. This service must be available 24 h per day and the team must include staff with the appropriate acute or critical care skills. The response should occur within a given timescale and alternative strategies must exist for when the maximum response time is exceeded
11 Develop and disseminate a DNACPR policy for the hospital. Identify patients who do not wish to be treated with CPR and those patients for whom cardiopulmonary arrest is an anticipated terminal event and in whom CPR is inappropriate
12 Audit cardiac arrests, "false arrests", unexpected deaths and unanticipated ICU admissions using common datasets. Audit the antecedents and clinical responses to these events

Further reading

Chan PS, Khalid A, Longmore LS, *et al.* Hospital-wide code rates and mortality before and after implementation of a rapid response team. *JAMA* 2008;**300**:2506–13.

Department of Health. *Competencies for Recognising and Responding to Acutely Ill Patients in Hospital.* London; 2009.

Featherstone P, Chalmers T, Smith GB. RSVP: a system for communication of deterioration in hospital patients. *Br J Nurs* 2008;**17**:860–4.

Meaney PA, Nadkarni VM, Kern KB, *et al.* Rhythms and outcomes of adult in-hospital cardiac arrest. *Crit Care Med* 2010;**38**:101–8.

National Early Warning Score (NEWS): Standardising the assessment of acute-illness severity in the NHS. Report of a working party. Royal College of Physicians, London; 2012.

Smith GB. In-hospital cardiac arrest: Is it time for an in-hospital 'chain of prevention'? *Resuscitation* 2010;**81**:1209–1211.

CHAPTER 4

Basic Life Support

Anthony J. Handley

Colchester Hospital University NHS Foundation Trust, Colchester, Essex, UK

OVERVIEW

- Early institution of CPR and defibrillation significantly increase the chance of survival after cardiac arrest
- Effective chest compression is vital, with correct depth and rate, and with a minimum of interruptions
- For the non-specialist, CPR on a child should follow the adult sequence of actions

---

Introduction

The term basic life support (BLS) is used to describe maintenance of a clear airway and support of breathing and the circulation in cases of cardiac arrest, without the use of equipment other than a simple airway device or protective shield. Cardiopulmonary resuscitation (CPR) is the combination of chest compression and rescue breathing, and forms the basis of modern BLS.

The chances of survival after cardiac arrest are increased when the event is witnessed and when a bystander institutes CPR prior to the arrival of the emergency services. When the heart arrests in ventricular fibrillation, the critical interval that determines outcome is the time from arrest until defibrillation, the chances of survival decreasing by between 7 and 10% for each minute of delay. Effective CPR reduces this decline by about 50%.

The best chance of a successful outcome for the patient is achieved if chest compressions are started as soon as cardiac arrest is diagnosed. Chest compressions should be given with minimal interruptions at the recommended rate and depth, and are accompanied by artificial ventilation according to the current guidelines (see Box 4.1 and Figure 4.1).

Box 4.1 **Optimal chest compression characteristics (adults)**

- Depth 5–6 cm
- Rate 100–120 min^{-1}
- Release pressure fully between each compression
- Minimise interruptions in CPR

ABC of Resuscitation, Sixth Edition. Edited by Jasmeet Soar, Gavin D. Perkins and Jerry Nolan.
© 2013 John Wiley & Sons, Ltd. Published 2013 by John Wiley & Sons, Ltd.

Diagnosing cardiac arrest

Although an absent carotid pulse in an unconscious patient is a sure sign of cardiac arrest, it has been shown that the accuracy of such a pulse check can be very poor, not only for laypeople. Unless the rescuer is trained, experienced, and confident in feeling for the carotid pulse, a diagnosis of cardiac arrest should be assumed if the patient is unresponsive and not breathing normally.

Agonal breathing

Particular care should be taken to recognise agonal breathing (irregular, often noisy, gasps) as a sign of cardiac arrest and not a sign of life. If agonal breathing is present, start CPR.

Circulatory support

A patient in cardiac arrest is unlikely to recover as a result of CPR alone, but rapid institution of resuscitation, particularly chest compression, can 'buy time' until a defibrillator and the emergency services arrive.

The correct place to compress the chest is in the centre of the lower half of the sternum. It is recommended that this location be taught in a simplified way, such as, 'place the heel of your hand in the centre of the chest with the other hand on top'. This instruction should be accompanied by a demonstration of placing the hands on the lower half of the sternum on a manikin. Use of the inter-nipple line as a landmark is not reliable.

Firm pressure is needed to compress the chest of an adult by 5–6 cm. The rescuer's arms should be kept straight with the elbows locked. About the same amount of time should be spent in the compressed phase as in the released phase, with complete release of pressure each time. The rate should be between 100–120 min^{-1} and compressions should be given in groups of 30, interspersed with 2 rescue breaths.

Ventilatory support

Establishing and maintaining an airway is the single most useful manoeuvre that the rescuer can perform. To open the airway, the patient's head should be tilted backwards (without hyperextension

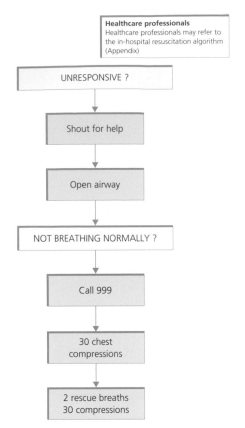

Healthcare professionals
Healthcare professionals may refer to
the in-hospital resuscitation algorithm
(Appendix)

UNRESPONSIVE ?

↓

Shout for help

↓

Open airway

↓

NOT BREATHING NORMALLY ?

↓

Call 999

↓

30 chest
compressions

↓

2 rescue breaths
30 compressions

Figure 4.1 Adult basic life support. Reproduced with the kind permission of the Resuscitation Council (UK).

of the neck) and the jaw lifted to pull the tongue forward off the posterior pharyngeal wall.

To give mouth-to-mouth ventilation the patient's nose should be pinched closed. The rescuer should then take a breath, make a firm seal with his or her lips around the patient's mouth, and breathe out, watching as the patient's chest clearly rises as in normal breathing. This should take about a second, and it is important to avoid over-inflation as this will allow air to enter the oesophagus and stomach. Subsequent gastric distension causes not only vomiting but also passive regurgitation into the lungs, which often goes undetected. The expired air is then allowed out passively. As soon as the chest falls, another breath should be given, with 30 chest compressions being given after every 2 rescue breaths.

Risks to rescuer and patient

The main concern during resuscitation is for the patient, but it is equally important to ensure that no harm comes to the rescuer.

Before approaching a collapsed patient, the rescuer should rapidly assess any personal danger as well as any to the patient from hazards such as falling masonry, gas, electricity, fire, or traffic.

Although there may be fears about catching HIV (human immunodeficiency virus), no case has been recorded due to mouth-to mouth-resuscitation. Despite the presence of the virus in saliva, it does not seem that transmission occurs via this route in the absence of blood-to-blood contact. There have been reports of the transmission of other infections, such as tuberculosis (TB) and

severe acute respiratory distress syndrome (SARS), but these have been very rare. Nevertheless, those who may be called upon to administer resuscitation should be allowed to use some form of barrier device, preferably a ventilation mask (for mouth-to-mask ventilation) or a filter device placed over the mouth and nose.

Adult basic life support sequence

Make sure the patient, any bystanders, and you are safe.
Check the patient for a response:

> Gently shake his shoulders and ask loudly, 'Are you all right?' (Figure 4.2)

If he responds:

> Leave him in the position in which you find him provided there is no further danger. Try to find out what is wrong with him and get help if needed
> Reassess him regularly

If he does not respond:

> Shout for help

Turn him onto his back and open the airway using head tilt and chin lift:

> Place your hand on his forehead and gently tilt his head back
> With your fingertips under the point of the patient's chin, lift the chin to open the airway (Figure 4.3)

Keeping the airway open, look, listen, and feel for normal breathing:

> Look for chest movement
> Listen at the patient's mouth for breath sounds
> Feel for air on your cheek (Figure 4.4)

Look, listen, and feel for no more than 10 seconds to determine if the patient is breathing normally. If you have any doubt whether breathing is normal, act as if it is not normal
If the patient is breathing normally:

> Turn him into the recovery (lateral) position (Figure 4.5)

If he is NOT breathing normally:

> Ask someone to call for an ambulance (or the emergency team if in hospital) and bring an AED if available. If you are on your own, use your mobile phone to call for an ambulance. Leave the patient only when no other option exists for getting help

Start chest compression as follows:

> Kneel by the side of the patient
> Place the heel of one hand in the centre of the patient's chest (which is the lower half of the patient's sternum)
> Place the heel of your other hand on top of the first hand
> Interlock the fingers of your hands and ensure that pressure is not applied over the patient's ribs. Do not apply any pressure over the upper abdomen or the bottom end of the sternum (Figure 4.6)
> Position yourself vertically above the patient's chest and, with your arms straight, press down on the sternum 5–6 cm (Figure 4.7)

After each compression, release all the pressure on the chest without losing contact between your hands and the sternum

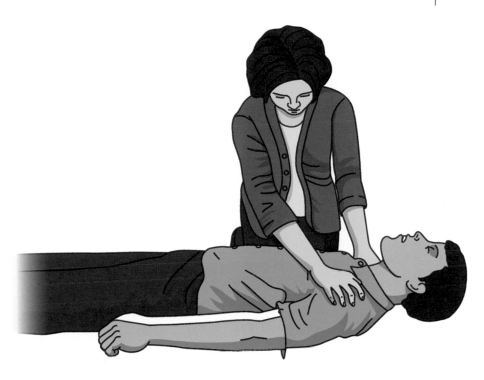

Figure 4.2 Establish responsiveness.

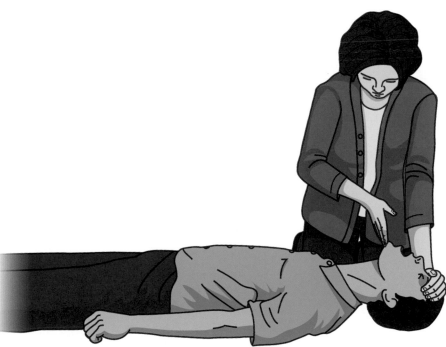

Figure 4.3 Head tilt – chin lift.

Repeat compressions at a rate of 100–120 min^{-1}

Compression and release should take an equal amount of time

Combine chest compression with rescue breaths:

After 30 compressions open the airway, again using head tilt and chin lift

Pinch the soft part of the patient's nose closed, using the index finger and thumb of your hand on his forehead

Allow his mouth to open, but maintain chin lift

Take a normal breath and place your lips around his mouth, making sure that you have a good seal (Figure 4.8)

Blow steadily into his mouth whilst watching for his chest to rise – take about one second to make his chest rise as in normal breathing: this is an effective rescue breath

Maintaining head tilt and chin lift, take your mouth away from the patient and watch for his chest to fall as air comes out

Take another normal breath and blow into the patient's mouth once more to give a total of two effective rescue breaths. The two breaths should not take more than 5 s. Then return your hands without delay to the correct position on the sternum and give a further 30 chest compressions

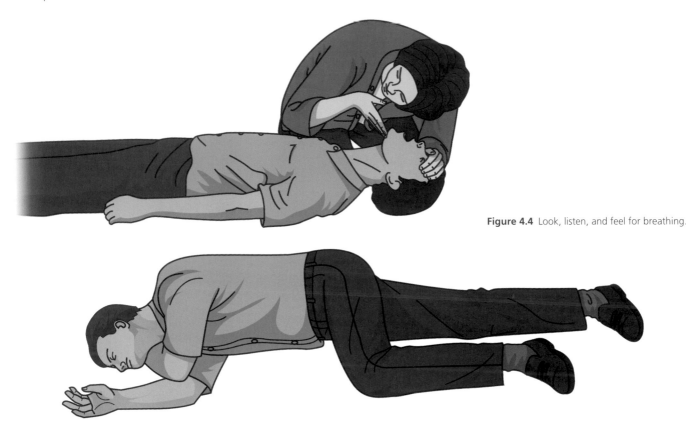

Figure 4.4 Look, listen, and feel for breathing.

Figure 4.5 Recovery (lateral) position.

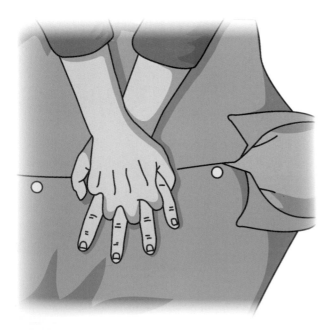

Figure 4.6 Hand position for chest compression.

Continue with chest compressions and rescue breaths in a ratio of 30:2

Stop to recheck the patient only if he starts to show signs of regaining consciousness, such as coughing, opening his eyes, speaking, or moving purposefully AND starts to breathe normally; otherwise do not interrupt resuscitation

Compression-only CPR

There is considerable published evidence that supports the concept of chest compression-only CPR for out-of-hospital cardiac arrest patients: it is simple and does not require rescuers to perform unpleasant mouth-to-mouth ventilation. The problem is that it is effective for a limited period only (probably less than 5 min) and, for a small but important minority of patients (children and those suffering an asphyxial or prolonged arrest), it is suboptimal treatment. It is not recommended as the standard management of out-of-hospital cardiac arrest, but should be considered (a) if the rescuer is untrained in CPR; (b) when an untrained rescuer is receiving telephone instruction from the ambulance dispatcher; (c) if the rescuer is unable or unwilling to perform rescue breathing.

CPR in children

Full details of resuscitation techniques for use in children will be found in Chapter 9. The following advice is for those who do not have a duty to respond to paediatric emergencies (usually health professional teams).

For ease of teaching and retention laypeople should be taught that the adult sequence may also be used for children (Figure 4.9) who are not responsive and not breathing.

Most laypeople taught CPR should perform the adult sequence on infants and children, BUT compress to one-third depth of chest. Physical damage following CPR in children is very rare. Therefore, do not be afraid that you may push too hard.

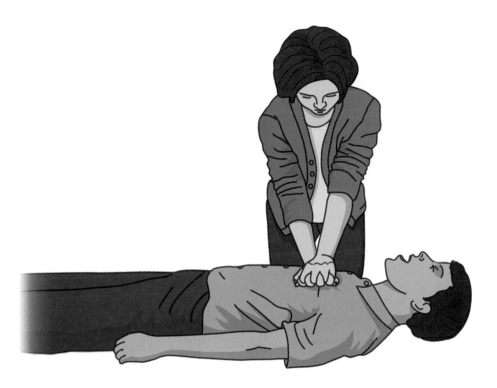

Figure 4.7 Compress the chest 5–6 cm at a rate of 100–120/min.

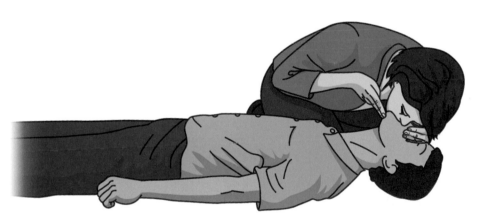

Figure 4.8 After 30 compressions give 2 rescue breaths.

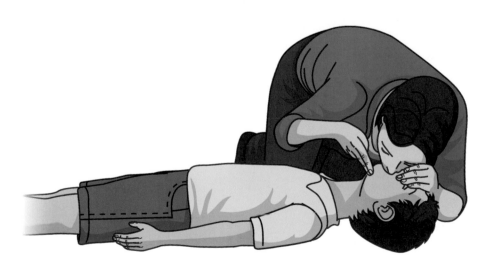

Figure 4.9 CPR in children.

Non-specialists, those laypeople who have responsibility for children (e.g. teachers, lifeguards, school nurses) or who are more likely to witness cardiac arrest in children (e.g. parents, child minders), and those who simply wish to extend their training may be taught to modify the adult sequence by (a) giving 5 initial breaths at the start of CPR, then continuing with a 30:2 compression:ventilation ratio; (b) compressing the child's chest to one-third its depth, using 2 fingers or 1 hand as appropriate to obtain the necessary depth; (c) performing CPR for about 1 min before leaving for help if this is necessary for a lone rescuer. If at all possible, training on a child manikin should be offered.

Further reading

Cardiopulmonary Resuscitation and Automated External Defibrillation (2nd edn), 2011. Resuscitation Council (UK), London.

Handley AJ, Colquhoun M. Adult BLS Guidelines In 2010 Resuscitation Guidelines. Resuscitation Council (UK). http://www.resus.org.uk/pages/bls.pdf

Koster RW, Baubin MA, Bossaert LL, Caballero A, Cassan P, Castrén M, *et al*. European Resuscitation Council Guidelines for Resuscitation 2010 Section 2. Adult basic life support and use of automated external defibrillators. *Resuscitation* 2010;**81**(10):1277–92.

CHAPTER 5

Advanced Life Support

Gavin D. Perkins[1], Jerry Nolan[2], Jasmeet Soar[3] and Susanna Price[4]

[1]Warwick Medical School, University of Warwick, UK
[2]Royal United Hospital, Bath, UK
[3]Southmead Hospital, North Bristol NHS, Bristol, UK
[4]Royal Brompton Hospital, London, UK

OVERVIEW

- The ALS algorithm summarises a series of advanced treatments for cardiac arrest
- Treatment is dictated by the patient's underlying heart rhythm
- First line treatment of shockable rhythms (ventricular fibrillation/ventricular tachycardia) is CPR and defibrillation
- First line treatment of non-shockable rhythms (pulseless electrical activity and asystole) is CPR, drugs and identification/treatment of reversible causes

---

Introduction

After cardiac arrest occurs, prompt and efficient action can be life saving. It is relatively rare for basic life support (BLS) interventions alone to restore a spontaneous circulation. Advanced life support (ALS) is the term used to describe a more extensive range of interventions, which includes advanced airway management, drugs, manual defibrillation, echocardiography, and identification and treatment of reversible causes of cardiac arrest. ALS interventions are usually provided by a team, for example an in-hospital resuscitation team or paramedic crew. Advanced life support algorithms facilitate team members working together in a structured and efficient manner enabling treatments to be given promptly without prolonged discussion.

ALS algorithm (Figure 5.1)

The first step in the ALS algorithm is to confirm cardiac arrest. The ALS provider is trained to check for breathing and feel for a pulse simultaneously. Cardiac arrest is confirmed by the absence of both a pulse and normal breathing; call the resuscitation team if not already present. Start high-quality, uninterrupted chest compressions and attach the patient to a defibrillator monitor with self-adhesive defibrillation/monitoring pads. Continue CPR by alternating 30 compressions with 2 ventilations until an advanced airway is inserted – this enables ventilation of the lungs without interrupting chest compressions. The underlying heart rhythm is assessed during

a coordinated, short pause in CPR; once the rhythm is confirmed, CPR is restarted whilst the next phase of treatment is planned.

The ALS algorithm provides two main treatment arms defined by the underlying heart rhythm (Figure 5.1). The main difference between the treatment arms is the requirement for defibrillation. Heart rhythms requiring defibrillation (ventricular fibrillation (VF) (Figure 5.2) or pulseless ventricular tachycardiac (VT)) are managed using the shockable side of the algorithm. Other rhythms (pulseless electrical activity (PEA) and asystole) are treated according to the non-shockable side of the algorithm.

Shockable rhythms (Box 5.1)

Prolonged interruptions in chest compressions before and after a shock are associated with reduced survival. Defibrillation attempts should minimise the peri-shock pauses to no more than a few seconds (see Chapter 6). Attempted defibrillation should be a coordinated sequence of actions (Figure 5.3). Once a shockable rhythm has been identified, restart chest compressions promptly. Charge the defibrillator to the appropriate energy level during chest compressions (150–200 J biphasic for the first shock and 150–360 J biphasic for subsequent shocks). Once the defibrillator is charged, all but the person performing chest compressions should stand clear of the patient. There is uncertainty about the safety of delivering a shock during manual chest compression, so once other members of the team are clear, the person performing chest compressions stops compressions and stands clear while the shock is delivered. Do not delay defibrillation by attempting to re-confirm the underlying rhythm prior to shock delivery. Once the shock is delivered, immediately restart chest compressions. Continue CPR for a further 2 min before pausing to reassess the heart rhythm.

Box 5.1 Treatment steps for shockable rhythms

- Plan actions before pausing CPR
- Pause CPR briefly and check rhythm
- Restart CPR
- If VF/VT present, charge defibrillator
- Team stand clear
- Stop compressions and stand clear
- Deliver shock
- Immediately resume CPR
- Continue CPR for 2 min before reassessing rhythm

ABC of Resuscitation, Sixth Edition. Edited by Jasmeet Soar, Gavin D. Perkins and Jerry Nolan.
© 2013 John Wiley & Sons, Ltd. Published 2013 by John Wiley & Sons, Ltd.

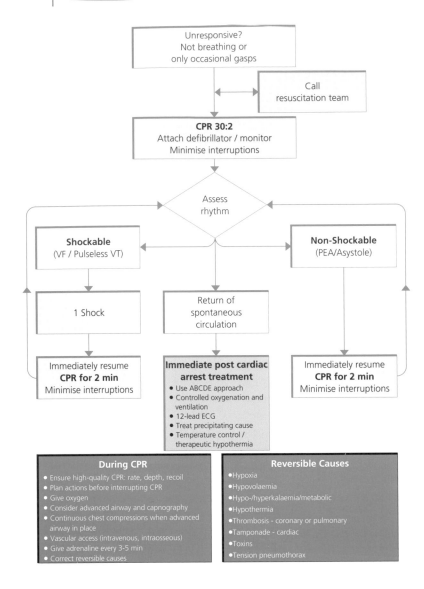

Figure 5.1 The adult Advanced Life Support Algorithm. Reproduced with the kind permission of the Resuscitation Council (UK).

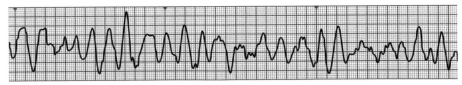

Figure 5.2 Ventricular Fibrillation (VF). Copyright 2012 Dr Oliver Meyer, Reproduced with permission.

If a shockable rhythm persists, repeat the shock sequence. Increase the energy level as indicated by the defibrillator manufacturer's instructions'. If a third shock is necessary, after shock delivery and restarting CPR, give adrenaline 1 mg and amiodarone 300 mg i.v. Further adrenaline 1 mg i.v may be given every 3–5 min thereafter (every other loop of the algorithm).

If during a rhythm check, organised electrical activity compatible with a cardiac output is seen, check for evidence of return of spontaneous circulation (ROSC). Signs of ROSC include a palpable pulse, spontaneous movements and/or a sudden increase in end-tidal carbon dioxide ($ETCO_2$) on waveform capnography. If ROSC has occurred, start post-resuscitation care. If there are no signs of ROSC, or if asystole or an agonal heart rhythm is seen during the rhythm check, continue CPR and switch over to the non-shockable algorithm.

Non-shockable rhythms (Box 5.2)

The non-shockable rhythms are PEA (organised electrical activity in the absence of a palpable pulse) and asystole (the absence of electrical activity). Survival from cardiac arrest with PEA or asystole is dependent on identifying and treating promptly a potentially reversible cause of the arrest.

Treatment for non-shockable rhythms focuses on high-quality, uninterrupted chest compression and identification and treatment of potentially reversible causes of the arrest (Table 5.1). Adrenaline (1 mg) increases the rate of ROSC and should be

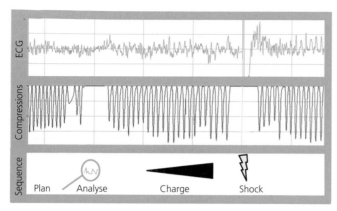

Figure 5.3 Defibrillation sequence. Plan actions; Pause CPR for rhythm analysis; Deliver shock; Restart CPR

given as soon as vascular access is available. Give further doses every 3–5 min (every other loop). Whether adrenaline improves long-term survival rates remains unknown.

Box 5.2 **Treatment steps for non-shockable rhythms**

- Provide high-quality chest compressions with minimal interrupts
- Give adrenaline 1 mg i.v./i.o.
- Attempt to identify reversible causes of cardiac arrest
- Continue CPR for 2 min before reassessing rhythm

Pause briefly to check the heart rhythm every 2 min. Unless there is evidence of ROSC, continue CPR. If a shockable rhythm is seen, switch to the shockable side of the algorithm.

During CPR (Box 5.3)

Ensure high-quality CPR is maintained throughout the resuscitation attempt. As soon as possible, obtain a definitive airway and vascular access. Look for evidence of potentially reversible causes of cardiac arrest (Table 5.1) and provide targeted treatment if appropriate. Give adrenaline 1 mg every 3–5 min.

Box 5.3 **During CPR**

- Continue high-quality CPR: ensure adequate depth, rate, full chest recoil
- Obtain a definitive airway
- Obtain vascular access
- Give drugs treatments as indicated
- Identify and treat reversible causes of cardiac arrest

High-quality CPR

Despite the quality of CPR being an important determinant of outcome, observational studies indicate that CPR is often poorly performed by healthcare professionals. Push hard and fast when doing CPR – aim for chest compression depths of 5–6 cm and rate of 100–120 min^{-1}. Remember when performing chest

Table 5.1 Potentially reversible causes of cardiac arrest and their treatment.

Cause	Indicators/tests	Treatment
Hypoxia	History Arterial blood gas analysis	High flow oxygen Secure the airway
Hypovolaemia	History Signs of bleeding Echocardiography / ultrasound	Stop haemorrhage Fluid resuscitation
Hyperkaleamia and electrolyte disturbances	History Laboratory tests Arterial blood gas analysis 12 lead ECG	Specific treatment targeted at correcting the specific electrolyte disturbance
Hypothermia	History Measure temperature	Warm IV fluids Invasive re-warming with cardiopulmonary bypass
Tension pneumothorax	Clinical signs Ultrasound	Chest decompression (thoracostomy or needle) Chest drain
Tamponade	History (penetrating chest injury, post cardiac surgery) Echocardiography	Pericardiocentesis Thoracotomy
Toxin	History	Specific treatment targeted at toxin (e.g. naloxone for opioid)
Thrombosis	History Clinical signs e.g. DVT Echocardiography/ultrasound	CPR Thrombolytic therapy

compressions with a patient on a mattress, you must push harder as the mattress will be compressed as well as the chest. Ensure that pressure on the chest is completely released between chest compressions. Avoid interruptions in chest compressions by pausing for no more than a few seconds during defibrillation and whilst securing an advanced airway. Once an advanced airway is in place, give continuous compressions (at $100–120\ \text{min}^{-1}$) while ventilating at $10\ \text{min}^{-1}$ without pausing the compressions.

Airway and ventilation

Tracheal intubation should be attempted only by trained staff with regular and ongoing experience of this technique (see Chapter 7). Confirm correct tube placement by direct vision, chest auscultation and waveform capnography. Unidentified misplacement of the tracheal tube will have catastrophic consequences. Supraglottic airway devices (e.g. laryngeal mask airway, I-gel or laryngeal tube) are an acceptable alternative to tracheal intubation. Ventilation of the lungs without pausing compressions is possible with supraglottic airway devices provided the leak is not excessive. Once the airway is secure, ventilate the lungs at approximately $10\ \text{ventilations min}^{-1}$. Avoid hyperventilation as this will reduce coronary perfusion pressure. As well as confirming correct tube placement, waveform capnography also enables monitoring of the quality of CPR and early identification of ROSC (visible as a sustained increase in in end tidal carbon dioxide).

Vascular access

Unless already available, obtain vascular access via the intravenous or intraosseous (IO) route. Peripheral venous cannulation is the safest route in an emergency. To enhance drug delivery to the central circulation, after injection of a drug, give a 20-ml bolus of fluid and elevate the limb. If rapid intravenous access cannot be obtained, consider the IO route (Figure 5.4). The IO route is safe and effective for fluid resuscitation and drug delivery in adults and children.

Drugs

No drug has been shown unequivocally to improve survival to discharge from cardiac arrest. Vasopressors such as adrenaline 1mg i.v. can improve the rate of ROSC and should be given every 3–5 min. Amiodarone 300mg i.v. has been shown to improve ROSC in VF arrest if given after initial defibrillation attempts are unsuccessful. Thromboloytic therapy is ineffective if given routinely when a cardiac cause of the arrest is suspected; however, very limited evidence suggests it may be effective as a treatment for massive pulmonary embolus. If thrombolytic therapy is given, continue CPR for at least 45 min. There is no evidence for the use of atropine during either asystole or PEA with slow a ventricular rate.

Ultrasound

In skilled hands, ultrasound can identify potentially reversible causes of cardiac arrest (Table 5.2). The use of ultrasound must not cause interruptions in CPR. Obtain cardiac images only when

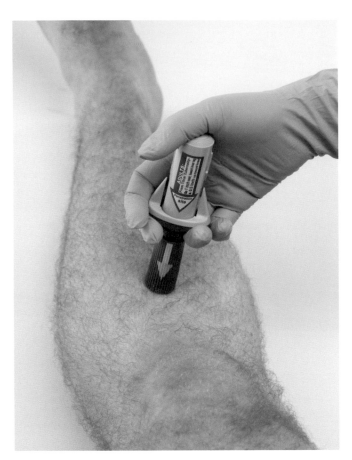

Figure 5.4 Methods for obtaining intraosseous access

CPR is stopped for planned pauses for rhythm checks and limit to less than 10 s. Training in Focused Echocardiogaphy Extended Life Support (FEEL) is recommended for this setting (http://www.feel-uk.com/).

Post-resuscitation care

If ROSC is obtained, start post-resuscitation care (see Chapter 8). Immediate steps comprise assessment and treatment of the patient using the ABCDE approach. Ensure adequate ventilation (normocapnia) and oxygenation (target SpO_2 94–98%). Obtain a 12-lead ECG to identify evidence of an acute coronary syndrome and consider early coronary reperfusion therapy. Start any specific treatment targeted at correcting the underlying cause of the arrest. Avoid hyperthermia and consider therapeutic hypothermia.

Stopping resuscitation and confirmation of death

More than half of all resuscitation attempts will fail to achieve ROSC. The decision to stop CPR requires a careful clinical assessment of the likelihood of the patient surviving if resuscitation attempts are continued. The cardiac arrest team leader should discuss and reach consensus with the rest of the resuscitation team before deciding to terminate resuscitation attempts.

Table 5.2 Ultrasound findings.

Pathology	Feature	Caveat
Tension pneumothorax	Ruled out if bilateral lung sliding demonstrated	In case of localised pneumothorax, need to evaluate multiple regions to exclude Absence of lung sliding does not diagnose pneumothorax
Pulmonary embolus	Dilated right heart Thrombus/mobile mass in right heart/ pulmonary trunk	Chronic pulmonary hypertension/cor pulmonale RV infarction Eustachian valve/prominent Chiari network
Hypovolaemia	Kissing left ventricular walls Small IVC (<1cm) at end expiration	Ventricular disease: may not be seen despite profound hypovolaemia/may be present despite euvolaemia in LVH Ventilated patient Large IVC does not correlate with volaemic status
Tamponade	Pericardial fluid collection Right ventricular diastolic collapse	Post-cardiac surgery may be misleading Haematoma in pericardial space may be difficult to identify
Other specific findings	Cardiac ischaemia: regional wall abnormalities Haemothorax: fluid in pleural cavity Abdominal aortic aneurysm: intimal tear, free fluid Aortic dissection: intimal tear, aortic incompetence Intra-abdominal bleeding: free fluid	May be seen in cardiomyopathy/myocarditis

After stopping CPR, death is confirmed after observing the patient for a minimum of 5 min and noting the absence of a central pulse on palpation and absence of heart sounds on auscultation. Additional tests for the confirmation of death are summarised in Box 5.4. The time and date of death and the name of the person confirming death should be recorded in the clinical record.

Box 5.4 Confirmation of death after CPR

- Observe for a minimum of 5 min after stopping CPR
- Confirm death through absence of central pulse and heart sounds
- Consider additional supporting signs:

  - Asystole on ECG monitor
  - Absence of pulsatile flow through arterial line
  - Absence of contractile activity using echocardiography

- After at least 5 min of continued cardiorespiratory arrest, confirm the absence of the pupillary responses to light, of the corneal reflexes, and of any motor response to supra-orbital pressure
- Document date and time of death and name of person confirming death

---

Informing the next of kin following a failed resuscitation attempt

Either a senior member of the resuscitation team or the patient's clinical team should inform the patient's next of kin after a failed resuscitation. Whenever possible this should be during a face-to-face meeting. The five Ps are a useful aide memoire for the steps involved in informing the next of kin after a sudden death (Box 5.5).

Box 5.5 Informing next of kin about death of a patient

- Prepare – review case notes to ensure thorough knowledge of events preceding death; identify an appropriate place to meet next of kin; find a colleague (doctors/nurse/paramedic) to accompany you, invite relatives to a face-to-face meeting
- Prompt – when next of kin arrives, respond promptly, do not keep them waiting
- Patient identity – confirm you are speaking to the relatives/next of kin of the deceased
- Provide information – do this sensitively and use unambiguous terms; check understanding
- Plans – explain what the next steps are likely to involve, e.g. coroner referral, death registration, funeral arrangements. Give written information leaflets when available

---

Further reading

Academy of Medical Royal Colleges. A code of practice for the diagnosis and confirmation of death. 2008. www.aomrc.org.uk

Deakin CD, Morrison LJ, Morley PT, *et al*. Advanced Life Support Chapter Collaborators. Part 8: Advanced life support: 2010 International Consensus on Cardiopulmonary Resuscitation and Emergency Cardiovascular Care Science with Treatment Recommendations. *Resuscitation* 2010;**81** (Suppl 1):e93–e174.

Deakin C, Nolan JP, Perkins GD, Lockey AS. Resuscitation Council (UK) Adult Advanced Life Support Guidelines. www.resus.org.uk/pages/als.pdf

Morley PT. Drugs during cardiopulmonary resuscitation. *Curr Opin Crit Care* 2011;**17**(3):214–8.

Perkins GD, Davies RP, Soar J, Thickett DR. The impact of manual defibrillation technique on no-flow time during simulated cardiopulmonary resuscitation. *Resuscitation* 2007;**73**:109–14.

CHAPTER 6

Defibrillation

Charles Deakin[1] and Michael Colquhoun[2]

[1]University Hospital Southampton, Southampton, UK
[2]Malvern, Worcestershire, UK

OVERVIEW

- Defibrillation is the definitive treatment of ventricular fibrillation/ventricular tachycardia (VF/VT) cardiac arrest
- Sufficient electric current must pass through the heart to abolish VF/VT
- The shorter the interval between the onset of VF/VT and delivery of the shock, the greater the chance of successful defibrillation and survival
- Chest compressions must be performed throughout resuscitation attempts, with interruptions for shocks kept to the minimum

Introduction

Defibrillation is the passage of sufficient electrical current across the heart to depolarise a critical mass of myocardium, preventing the continued propagation of the fibrillatory wave fronts and allowing the natural pacemaker in the heart to resume control of the cardiac rhythm. Following the onset of VF or VT, cardiac output ceases and cerebral hypoxic injury rapidly ensues. For recovery to be possible, defibrillation with the return of a spontaneous circulation (ROSC) must be achieved as soon as possible.

Untreated, VF decays into terminal asystole as cardiac energy sources become exhausted; this process can be slowed by effective CPR. The probability of successful defibrillation declines rapidly with time: for every minute that passes between collapse and attempted defibrillation, the chance of success declines by approximately 10%.

Defibrillators

All defibrillators have features in common: a power source capable of providing electric current, a capacitor that can be charged to a pre-determined energy level and two electrodes which are placed on the patient's chest, either side of the heart, across which the capacitor is discharged. The electrodes may also act as monitoring electrodes for the ECG rhythm.

ABC of Resuscitation, Sixth Edition. Edited by Jasmeet Soar, Gavin D. Perkins and Jerry Nolan.
© 2013 John Wiley & Sons, Ltd. Published 2013 by John Wiley & Sons, Ltd.

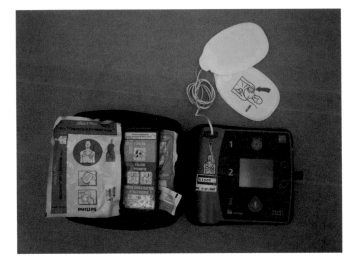

Figure 6.1 Example of an automatic external defibrillator. Reproduced by permission of Professor Charles Deakin. Copyright © 2012 Charles Deakin.

With manual defibrillators, the operator interprets the ECG and has to decide if the rhythm is one likely to respond to a shock. This requires skill and training requirements are therefore increased.

With automated external defibrillators (AEDs; Figure 6.1) voice prompts and instructions on a screen direct the operator through the procedure. ECG analysis is automated and the machine charges and directs the operator to deliver the shock if appropriate. Modern devices are highly accurate and reliable and it is almost impossible to deliver a shock inappropriately. Prompts to perform CPR are also given. Training in the use of AEDs can be achieved much more rapidly and easily than for manual defibrillators and has extended dramatically the range of personnel who can defibrillate.

The reliability of modern AEDs has made the concept of public access defibrillation (PAD) a reality. AEDs are placed in areas of high risk (transport and sporting facilities in particular) and are used by trained laypeople working nearby to provide defibrillation prior to ambulance arrival. Survival rates of up to 74% have been reported under optimal circumstances.

Factors influencing defibrillation

Transthoracic impedance

The success of attempted defibrillation depends on sufficient current being delivered to the myocardium. The major determinant of

Table 6.1 Factors affecting transthoracic impedance.

Chest size/inter-electrode distance	Larger chest = higher impedance
The energy of the shock	Higher energies reduce impedance
Electrode size	Larger electrodes reduce impedance
Electrode and chest wall interface	Couplants (gels/pastes) lower impedance
	Shaving hairy chests improves contact
Phase of ventilation	Lower at end-expiration
Number of shocks	Impedance falls with successive shocks
Electrode pressure	Firm pressure lowers impedance

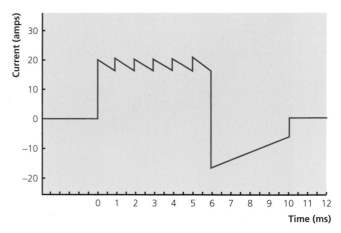

Figure 6.3 Biphasic rectilinear waveform. Reproduced from Deakin CD, Nolan JP, Sunde K, Koster RW. European Resuscitation Council Guidelines for Resuscitation 2010. Section 3: Electrical therapies. Resuscitation 2010;81:1293–1304. Copyright 2010, Elsevier.

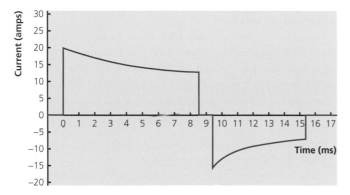

Figure 6.2 Biphasic truncated exponential waveform. Reproduced from Deakin CD, Nolan JP, Sunde K, Koster RW. European Resuscitation Council Guidelines for Resuscitation 2010. Section 3: Electrical therapies. Resuscitation 2010;81:1293–1304. Copyright 2010, Elsevier.

current flow is the electrical resistance presented by the thorax, the transthoracic impedance, which in adults is normally in the range 70–80 Ohm. Defibrillation technique must be optimised to minimise this transthoracic impedance thereby maximising the current delivered to the myocardium.

Transthoracic impedance can be influenced by various factors as outlined in Table 6.1.

Modern biphasic defibrillators measure transthoracic impedance immediately prior to shock delivery and adjust the energy delivered to compensate and are therefore less susceptible to higher transthoracic impedance (impedance compensation).

Shock waveform

Biphasic defibrillators deliver current that flows in a positive direction for a specified duration before reversing polarity to a negative direction for the remainder of the electrical discharge. There are two main types of biphasic waveform: the biphasic truncated exponential (BTE; Figure 6.2) and the rectilinear biphasic (RLB; Figure 6.3); there is no evidence that either is more effective than the other.

Biphasic waveforms are more effective at terminating both atrial and ventricular arrhythmias at lower energy levels and have a greater first-shock efficacy than the older monophasic waveforms, particularly for long duration VF/VT (85–98% compared with 54–91%). Hence the use of biphasic waveforms is recommended whenever possible. All new defibrillators deliver shocks with biphasic waveforms.

Shock energy

The optimal energy levels for defibrillation are unknown and the recommendations below are based on a consensus following a review of the current scientific literature. The aim is to achieve defibrillation and ROSC while minimising myocardial injury by using the lowest effective energy and reducing the number of repetitive shocks.

The initial biphasic shock energy is 150 J, irrespective of the biphasic waveform. If the provider is unaware of the type of defibrillator (monophasic or biphasic) or its effective dose range, use the highest available energy for the first and all subsequent shocks. If the first shock is unsuccessful, second and subsequent shocks can be delivered using either fixed or escalating energies of between 150 and 360 J, depending on the device. If a shockable rhythm recurs after successful defibrillation (with or without ROSC), give the next shock with the energy level that had previously been successful.

When using a monophasic defibrillator, use 360 J for the first and all subsequent shocks.

Shock sequence

With first-shock efficacy of biphasic waveforms generally exceeding 90%, failure to cardiovert VF successfully suggests the need for a period of CPR to perfuse the myocardium, rather than a further shock. Subsequently, a 2005 guidelines change to single shocks rather than three stacked shocks has demonstrated improved defibrillation success and increased survival to hospital discharge. Even if the defibrillation attempt is successful in restoring a perfusing rhythm, it is very rare for a pulse to be palpable immediately after defibrillation. Therefore, irrespective of the outcome of the shock, resume CPR for 2 min before reassessing the rhythm and performing a pulse check (see Chapter 5).

Electrode position

Recommended electrode positions are those that are believed to result in the highest current density through the heart, particularly important since no more than 4% of total delivered energy crosses the myocardium.

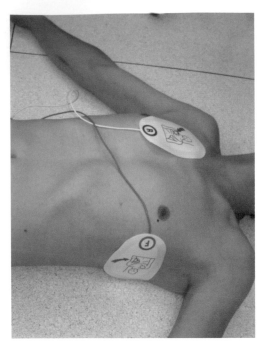

Figure 6.4 Antero-lateral self-adhesive pad position. Reproduced by permission of Professor Charles Deakin. Copyright © 2012 Charles Deakin.

Acceptable pad positions include:

- *Antero-lateral*: One electrode to the right of the sternum, immediately below the clavicle; the other placed in the mid-axillary line, approximately level with the V6 ECG electrode, clear of any breast tissue (Figure 6.4).
- *Antero-posterior*: One electrode anteriorly, over the left precordium, and the other electrode on the back behind the heart, medial to the left scapula (antero-posterior).
- *Bi-axillary*: Each electrode on the lateral chest walls, one on the right and the other on the left side.

Chest compressions

Continuous, uninterrupted chest compressions optimise the chance of successful defibrillation. Even short interruptions in chest compressions (to deliver rescue breaths or perform rhythm analysis) significantly reduce the chances of successful defibrillation. Analysis of CPR performance during out-of-hospital and in-hospital cardiac arrest has shown that significant interruptions are common and every effort should be made to minimise these. The aim should be to ensure that chest compressions are performed continuously throughout the resuscitation attempt, only pausing briefly to enable specific interventions.

The duration of the interval between stopping chest compressions and delivering the shock, the pre-shock pause, is also an important factor. The chance of successful defibrillation decreases as the pre-shock pause lengthens; every 5-s increase almost halves the chance of successful defibrillation. Consequently, defibrillation must always be performed quickly and efficiently, thus maximising the chance of successful resuscitation.

Safety

Accidental electrocution

Attempted defibrillation should be undertaken without risk to members of the resuscitation team. This is achieved best by using self-adhesive pad electrodes as this reduces the risk of accidental contact with the electrode. The operator must ensure that everyone is clear of the patient and attached equipment before delivering a shock. Gloves may provide some protection from the electric current; therefore it is strongly recommended that all members of the resuscitation team wear gloves.

Safe use of oxygen

Sparking from poorly applied defibrillator paddles in an oxygen-enriched atmosphere has caused fires and many have resulted in significant burns to the patient. The use of self-adhesive pads is far less likely to cause sparks than manual paddles – no fires have been reported in association with the use of self-adhesive pads. The following are recommended as good practice:

- Remove any oxygen mask or nasal cannulae and place them at least 1 m away from the patient's chest.
- Leave the ventilation bag (Figure 6.5) connected to the tracheal tube or supraglottic airway device; no increase in oxygen concentration occurs in the zone of defibrillation, even with an oxygen flow of $15 \, l \, min^{-1}$. Alternatively, disconnect the ventilation bag and remove it at least 1 m from the patient's chest during defibrillation.

Cardiac pacemakers and implantable cardioverter-defibrillators (ICD)

Be careful if the patient has a cardiac pacemaker or implantable cardioverter-defibrillator (ICD) because the current may travel along the pacemaker wire or ICD lead causing burns where the electrode tip makes contact with the myocardium. Place the defibrillator electrodes at least 8 cm from the pacemaker unit to minimise

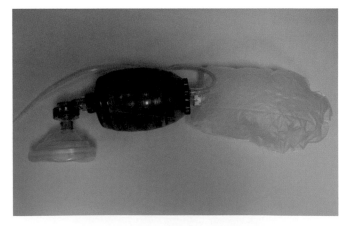

Figure 6.5 Remove the ventilation bag and mask at least 1 m away from the patient. Reproduced by permission of Professor Charles Deakin. Copyright © 2012 Charles Deakin.

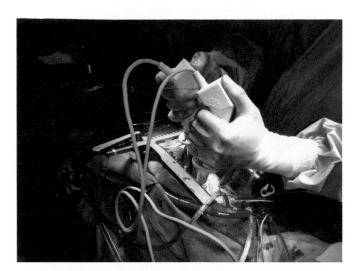

Figure 6.6 Internal cardioversion being performed during cardiac surgery. Reproduced by permission of Professor Charles Deakin. Copyright © 2012 Charles Deakin.

this risk, using the antero-posterior or postero-lateral position as necessary. If resuscitation is successful, the pacemaker threshold and generator will need to be checked.

Recent case reports have documented rescuers receiving shocks from ICD devices when in contact with the patient during CPR. It is particularly important to wear gloves and avoid skin-to-skin contact with the patient while performing CPR as there is no warning before the ICD discharges.

Internal defibrillation

Internal defibrillation using paddles applied directly across the ventricles (Figure 6.6) requires considerably less energy than that used for external defibrillation. Again, biphasic shocks using 10–20 J are substantially more effective than monophasic shocks.

Further reading

Deakin CD. Advances in Defibrillation. *Current Opinion in Critical Care* 2011;**17**:231–5.

Deakin CD, Nolan JP, Soar J, *et al*. European Resuscitation Council Guidelines for Resuscitation 2010. Section 4: Adult advanced life support. *Resuscitation* 2010;**81**:1305–52.

Deakin CD, Nolan JP, Sunde K, Koster RW. European Resuscitation Council Guidelines for Resuscitation 2010. Section 3: Electrical therapies. *Resuscitation* 2010;**81**:1293–304.

Kerber RE, Deakin CD, Tacker WA. Transthoracic defibrillation. In *Cardiac arrest. The Science and Practice of Resuscitation Medicine* (2nd edn), Chapter 25 (eds Paradis NA, Halperin HR, Kern KB *et al*.), Cambridge University Press, 2007.

CHAPTER 7

Airway Management and Ventilation

Jerry Nolan[1] and Jasmeet Soar[2]

[1]Royal United Hospital, Bath, UK
[2]Southmead Hospital, North Bristol NHS Trust, Bristol, UK

OVERVIEW

- Airway patency and ventilating the lungs are important components of CPR
- Simple airway manoeuvres, with or without basic adjuncts, will often achieve a patent airway
- Give all patients high concentration oxygen until the arterial oxygen saturation is measurable
- Supraglottic airway devices (SADs) are good alternatives to the bag-mask and should be used instead of the bag-mask technique wherever possible
- SADs should be used instead of tracheal intubation unless individuals highly skilled in intubation are immediately available
- When undertaken by someone with appropriate skills and experience, tracheal intubation is an effective airway management technique during cardiopulmonary resuscitation
- In unskilled hands, prolonged interruptions of chest compressions, and the high risk of failure and other complications (e.g. unrecognised oesophageal intubation) make tracheal intubation attempts potentially harmful
- Waveform capnography should be used whenever tracheal intubation is attempted

---

Introduction

Patients requiring resuscitation often have an obstructed airway, usually caused by loss of consciousness, but occasionally it may be the primary cause of cardiorespiratory arrest. Immediate restoration of airway patency enables ventilation of the lungs and oxygenation of the blood. Without adequate oxygenation it may be impossible to restore a perfusing cardiac rhythm. There is little high-quality evidence to support the use of any specific technique for maintaining an airway in adults with cardiorespiratory arrest. Ventilation is often achieved using a self-inflating bag and a mask ('bag-mask'), but use of supraglottic airway devices (SADs) may be more effective and reduce the risk of gastric inflation. Tracheal intubation is generally considered to be the optimal method for maintaining a clear

ABC of Resuscitation, Sixth Edition. Edited by Jasmeet Soar, Gavin D. Perkins and Jerry Nolan.

airway but it should be attempted only when trained personnel are available to carry out the procedure with a high level of skill and competence.

Causes of airway obstruction

Airway obstruction may be partial or complete. It can occur at any level from the nose and mouth down to the level of the carina and bronchi. In unconscious patients, the commonest site of airway obstruction is at the soft palate and epiglottis and, contrary to popular belief, not the tongue. Vomit or blood, as a result of regurgitation of gastric contents or trauma, or foreign bodies can also cause airway obstruction. Laryngeal obstruction may be caused by oedema from burns, inflammation or anaphylaxis. Upper airway stimulation or inhalation of foreign material may cause laryngeal spasm. Obstruction of the airway below the larynx is less common, but may be caused by excessive bronchial secretions, mucosal oedema, bronchospasm, pulmonary oedema, or aspiration of gastric contents. Extrinsic compression of the airway may also occur above or below the larynx, for example as a result of trauma, haematoma or tumour.

Recognition of airway obstruction

Airway obstruction can be subtle. Use the look, listen and feel approach:

- LOOK for chest and abdominal movements
- LISTEN and FEEL for airflow at the mouth and nose

In partial airway obstruction, air entry is diminished and usually noisy: inspiratory stridor is caused by obstruction at the laryngeal level or above; expiratory wheeze suggests obstruction of the lower airways, which tend to collapse and obstruct during expiration.

Complete airway obstruction in a patient who is making respiratory efforts causes paradoxical chest and abdominal movement, described as 'see-saw breathing'. During airway obstruction, accessory muscles of respiration are used; there may also be intercostal and subcostal recession and a tracheal tug.

During apnoea, when spontaneous breathing movements are absent, complete airway obstruction is recognised by failure to inflate the lungs during attempted positive pressure ventilation. Airway obstruction must be relieved rapidly otherwise brain

Table 7.1 Signs and symptoms of mild and severe airway obstruction.

General signs of choking	Attack occurs while eating Patient may clutch his neck	
Signs of airway obstruction	Mild	Severe
Response to question 'Are you choking?'	Speaks and answers yes	Unable to speak May respond by nodding
Other signs	Able to speak, cough and breathe	Unable to breathe Breathing sounds wheezy Attempts at coughing are silent May be unconscious

Adult Choking Treatment Algorithm

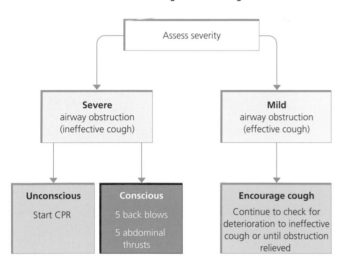

Figure 7.1 Adult choking algorithm. Reproduced with the kind permission of the Resuscitation Council (UK).

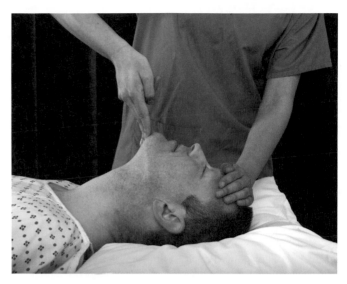

Figure 7.2 Head tilt and chin lift. Photograph reproduced with kind permission by Michael Scott and the Resuscitation Council (UK).

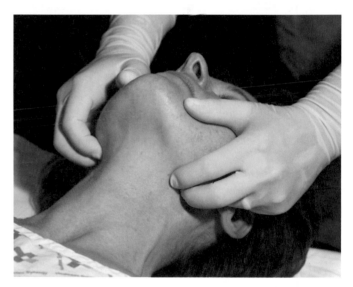

Figure 7.3 Jaw thrust. Photograph reproduced with kind permission by Michael Scott and the Resuscitation Council (UK).

injury will start to occur within a few minutes. Initially, give high concentration oxygen during attempts to relieve airway obstruction: as airway patency improves, arterial blood oxygen saturation (SaO_2) levels will be restored more rapidly if the inspired oxygen concentration is initially high.

Choking

Foreign bodies can cause either mild or severe airway obstruction. The signs and symptoms of mild and severe airway obstruction are summarised in Table 7.1. The appropriate treatment is shown in the adult choking algorithm (Figure 7.1).

Basic techniques for opening the airway

The head tilt, chin lift (Figure 7.2) and jaw thrust (Figure 7.3) can be used to relieve upper airway obstruction.

Airway manoeuvres in a patient with suspected cervical spine injury

If spinal injury is suspected, the head, neck, chest and lumbar region are maintained in the neutral position during resuscitation. When there is a risk of cervical spine injury, establish a clear upper airway by using jaw thrust or chin lift in combination with manual in-line stabilisation (MILS) of the head and neck by an assistant. Establishing a patent airway takes priority over concerns about a potential cervical spine injury.

Adjuncts to basic airway techniques

Oropharyngeal and nasopharyngeal airways will overcome soft palate obstruction and backward tongue displacement in an unconscious patient, but head tilt and jaw thrust may also be required.

The appropriate size for an oropharyngeal airway corresponds to the vertical distance between the patient's incisors and the angle of the jaw. In patients who are not deeply unconscious, a nasopharyngeal airway is better tolerated than an oropharyngeal airway; sizes 6–7 mm are suitable for adults.

Oxygen

During CPR, the lungs are ventilated with 100% oxygen until return of a spontaneous circulation (ROSC) is achieved. After ROSC is achieved, high-flow oxygen is given until the SaO_2 can be measured reliably. There are animal data indicating an association between high SaO_2 (hyperoxaemia) after ROSC and worse outcome. Clinical data from observational studies are conflicting but the current recommendations are that when blood oxygen saturation can be measured reliably, oxygen saturations should be maintained between 94 and 98%; or between 88 and 92% if the patient has chronic obstructive pulmonary disease.

Ventilation

Expired air ventilation (rescue breathing) is effective but the rescuer's expired oxygen concentration is only 16–17%, so it must be replaced as soon as possible by ventilation with oxygen-enriched air. The pocket resuscitation mask is similar to an anaesthetic face mask and enables mouth-to-mask ventilation. It has a unidirectional valve, which directs the patient's expired air away from the rescuer. Some masks have a port for the addition of oxygen. When using masks without an oxygen port, supplemental oxygen can be given by placing oxygen tubing underneath one side and ensuring an adequate seal. Tidal volumes in the region of $6–7\,ml\,kg^{-1}$ will provide adequate oxygenation and ventilation, while minimising the risk of gastric inflation. Each breath is delivered over approximately 1 s and to a volume that corresponds to normal visible chest movement. During CPR with an unprotected airway, give 2 ventilations after every 30 chest compressions.

Self-inflating bag

The self-inflating bag can be connected to a face mask, tracheal tube, or supraglottic airway device. When used with supplemental oxygen and a reservoir system (usually standard on modern devices) an inspired oxygen concentration of approximately 85% is achieved. Although the bag-mask apparatus enables ventilation with high concentrations of oxygen, its use by a single person requires considerable skill; therefore, the two-person technique is preferable (Figure 7.4).

Supraglottic airway devices

In comparison with bag-mask ventilation, use of SADs may enable more effective ventilation and reduce the risk of gastric inflation. They are also easier to insert than a tracheal tube and can generally be positioned without interrupting chest compressions. Alternative airway devices should be used by those unskilled in tracheal intubation or if a skilled operator is unable intubate.

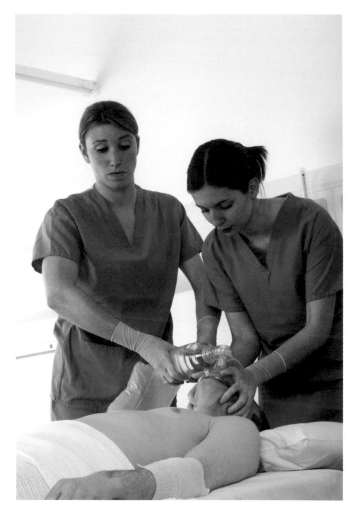

Figure 7.4 Two-person technique for bag-mask ventilation. Photograph reproduced with kind permission by Michael Scott and the Resuscitation Council (UK).

Laryngeal mask airway (LMA)

Effective use of the LMA by nursing, paramedical and medical staff during resuscitation has been documented, although these are generally observational studies. The need to resterilise the reusable LMA Classic™ make single-use LMAs more suitable for resuscitation. Some single-use LMAs are of a slightly different design and material to the LMA Classic™ and their performance has not been validated in the CPR setting.

In the presence of high airway resistance or poor lung compliance there is a risk of hypoventilation caused by a significant leak around the cuff. Attempt continuous compressions initially but abandon this if persistent leaks and hypoventilation occur.

The ProSeal LMA

The ProSeal LMA (PLMA) is a modified LMA: it has an additional posterior cuff, a gastric drain tube (enabling venting of liquid regurgitated gastric contents from the upper oesophagus and passage of a gastric tube to drain liquid gastric contents), and incorporates a bite block. There are no studies of its performance

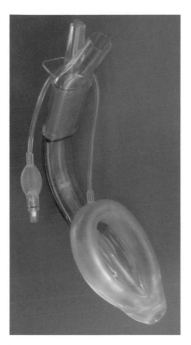

Figure 7.5 LMA Supreme.

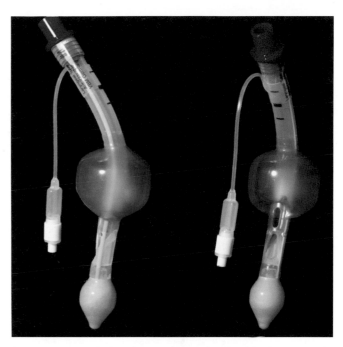

Figure 7.7 Laryngeal tube. Photograph reproduced with kind permission by Michael Scott and the Resuscitation Council (UK).

during CPR but it enables ventilation at higher airway pressures (up to 35–40 cmH$_2$O), which may enable adequate ventilation during uninterrupted chest compressions. A disposable version, the LMA Supreme (Figure 7.5), may be ideally suited to CPR but has yet to be studied for this purpose.

I-gel airway

The I-gel has a preformed cuff that does not require inflation. The stem of the I-gel incorporates a bite block and a narrow oesophageal drain tube (Figure 7.6). Its ease of insertion and favourable leak pressure (20–24 cmH$_2$O) make it theoretically very attractive as

a resuscitation airway device for those inexperienced in tracheal intubation. Use of the I-gel during cardiac arrest has been reported but more data on its use in this setting are awaited.

Laryngeal tube

The laryngeal tube (LT) is a single-lumen tube with both an oesophageal and pharyngeal cuff (Figure 7.7). A single pilot balloon inflates both cuffs simultaneously and it is available in a variety of sizes. There are several observational studies that document successful use of the LT by nurses and paramedics during prehospital cardiac arrest. A double lumen LT with an oesophageal vent and a disposable version (LT-D) are available.

Tracheal intubation

Tracheal intubation should be used only when trained personnel are available to carry out the procedure with a high level of skill and competence. No study has shown improved outcome with tracheal intubation after cardiac arrest; indeed, several observational studies document an association between tracheal intubation and worse outcome.

The perceived advantages of tracheal intubation over bag-mask ventilation include maintenance of a patent airway which is protected from aspiration of gastric contents or blood from the oropharynx, ability to provide an adequate tidal volume reliably even when chest compressions are uninterrupted, the potential to free the rescuer's hands for other tasks and the ability to suck-out airway secretions. Use of a bag-mask is more likely to cause gastric distension, which, theoretically, is more likely to cause regurgitation and the risk of aspiration. This theoretical risk has yet to be proven in randomised clinical trials.

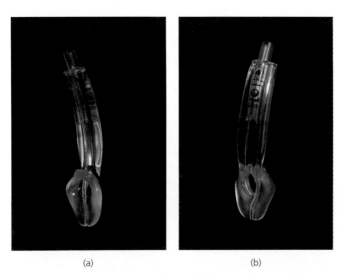

(a)   (b)

Figure 7.6 I-gel. Photograph reproduced with kind permission by Michael Scott and the Resuscitation Council (UK).

The perceived disadvantages of tracheal intubation over bag-mask ventilation include the risk of an unrecognised misplaced tracheal tube (up to 17% in some out-of-hospital cardiac arrest studies), a prolonged time without chest compressions while tracheal intubation is attempted (for almost 25% of all CPR interruptions in one study) and a comparatively high failure rate. In one study involving pre-hospital intubation of 100 cardiac arrest patients by paramedics, the first intubation attempt accounted for a median interruption in CPR of 45 s and in one third of cases it exceeded 1 min.

Personnel skilled in advanced airway management should be able to undertake laryngoscopy without stopping chest compressions; a brief pause in chest compressions will be required only as the tube is passed through the vocal cords. Alternatively, to avoid any interruptions in chest compressions, the intubation attempt may be deferred until return of spontaneous circulation (ROSC). No tracheal intubation attempt should interrupt chest compressions for more than 10 s; if intubation is not achievable within these constraints, recommence bag-mask or bag-SAD ventilation. After tracheal intubation, tube placement must be confirmed and the tube secured adequately. If there is any doubt about the correct position of the tube, remove it and re-oxygenate the patient before making another attempt.

Confirmation of correct tracheal tube placement

Unrecognised oesophageal intubation is the most serious complication of attempted tracheal intubation. Routine use of primary and secondary techniques to confirm correct placement of the tracheal tube will reduce this risk.

Clinical assessment

Primary assessment includes observation of chest expansion bilaterally, auscultation over the lung fields bilaterally in the axillae and over the epigastrium. Secondary confirmation of tracheal tube placement by an exhaled carbon dioxide (CO_2) or oesophageal detection device should reduce the risk of unrecognised oesophageal intubation but the performance of the available devices varies considerably.

Oesophageal detector device

The oesophageal detector device creates a suction force at the tracheal end of the tracheal tube, either by pulling back the plunger on a large syringe or releasing a compressed flexible bulb. Air is aspirated easily from the lower airways through a tracheal tube placed in the cartilage-supported rigid trachea. When the tube is in the oesophagus, air cannot be aspirated because the oesophagus collapses when aspiration is attempted. The oesophageal detector device may be misleading in patients with morbid obesity, late pregnancy or severe asthma or when there are copious tracheal secretions; in these conditions the trachea may collapse when aspiration is attempted.

Carbon dioxide detectors

Unless cardiac arrest has been very prolonged (more than 30 min), chest compressions will produce sufficient pulmonary blood flow to produce detectable exhaled CO_2 concentrations. Following a tracheal intubation attempt, if exhaled CO_2 is not detected, assume the tube is in the oesophagus.

Carbon dioxide detector devices measure the concentration of exhaled carbon dioxide from the lungs; there are broadly three types:

1 Disposable colorimetric end-tidal carbon dioxide ($ETCO_2$) detectors use a litmus paper to detect CO_2, and these devices generally give readings of purple ($ETCO_2 < 0.5\%$), tan ($ETCO_2$ 0.5–2%) and yellow ($ETCO_2 > 2\%$)
2 Non-waveform electronic digital $ETCO_2$ devices measure $ETCO_2$ using an infrared spectrometer and display the results with a number
3 End-tidal CO_2 detectors that include a waveform graphical display (capnograph) are the most reliable for verification of tracheal tube position during cardiac arrest. Studies of waveform capnography to verify tracheal tube position in victims of cardiac arrest demonstrate 100% sensitivity and 100% specificity in identifying correct tracheal tube placement

Waveform capnography is the most sensitive and specific way to confirm and continuously monitor the position of a tracheal tube in victims of cardiac arrest but will not discriminate between tracheal and bronchial placement of the tube – careful auscultation is essential. Existing portable monitors make capnographic initial confirmation and continuous monitoring of tracheal tube position feasible in almost all settings, including out-of-hospital, emergency department and in-hospital locations where tracheal intubation is performed. Waveform capnography is also a sensitive indicator of ROSC. The current standard is that tracheal intubation should not be undertaken unless waveform capnography is available.

Cricothyroidotomy

Occasionally it will be impossible to ventilate an apnoeic patient with a bag-mask, or to pass a tracheal tube or other airway device. This may occur in patients with extensive facial trauma or laryngeal obstruction caused by oedema (e.g. anaphylaxis). In these circumstances, a surgical cricothyroidotomy provides a definitive airway that can be used to ventilate the patient's lungs until semi-elective intubation or tracheostomy is performed. Needle cricothyroidotomy is a much more temporary procedure providing only short-term oxygenation. It requires a wide-bore, non-kinking cannula, a high-pressure oxygen source and may cause serious barotrauma. It is also prone to failure because of kinking of the cannula, and is unsuitable for patient transfer.

The Royal College of Anaesthetists and Difficult Airway Society National Audit Project 4 (NAP4) documented a high failure rate (60%) when airway rescue was attempted with needle cricothyroidotomy. In contrast, all surgical cricothyroidotomies achieved access to the trachea.

Further reading

Deakin CD, Morrison LJ, Morley PT, *et al.* 2010 International Consensus on Cardiopulmonary Resuscitation and Emergency Cardiovascular Care Science with Treatment Recommendations. Part 8: Advanced Life Support. *Resuscitation* 2010;**81**(Suppl 1):e93–e174.

Deakin CD, Nolan JP, Soar J, *et al.* European Resuscitation Council Guidelines for Resuscitation 2010. Section 4. Adult advanced life support. *Resuscitation* 2010;**81**:1305–52.

Nolan JP, Kelly FE. Airway challenges in critical care. *Anaesthesia* 2011;**66**(Suppl 2):81–92.

Nolan JP, Soar J. Airway techniques and ventilation strategies. *Curr Opin Crit Care* 2008;**14**:279–86.

Wang HE, Simeone SJ, Weaver MD, Callaway CW. Interruptions in cardiopulmonary resuscitation from paramedic endotracheal intubation. *Ann Emerg Med* 2009;**54**:645–52.

CHAPTER 8

Post-Resuscitation Care

Jerry Nolan

Royal United Hospital, Bath, UK

OVERVIEW

- The treatment a patient receives after return of spontaneous circulation influences significantly the ultimate outcome
- The post-cardiac arrest syndrome impacts particularly the brain and cardiovascular system but the ischaemia/reperfusion response can affect all organs
- Targeted temperature management and, where appropriate, percutaneous coronary intervention are two key post-cardiac arrest interventions
- Predicating the outcome for the comatose post-cardiac arrest patient remains challenging

---

Introduction

Return of a spontaneous circulation (ROSC) is a critical step in the continuum of resuscitation, but the quality of the patient's ultimate survival depends on interventions applied in the post-resuscitation phase – the final link in the chain of survival. Post-resuscitation treatment starts at the location where ROSC is achieved but, once stabilised, the patient is transferred to the most appropriate high-care area (e.g. intensive care unit (ICU), coronary care unit (CCU)) for continued monitoring and treatment.

The post-cardiac arrest syndrome

Components of the post-cardiac arrest syndrome are shown in Box 8.1.

Box 8.1 **Components of the post-cardiac arrest syndrome**

- Post-cardiac arrest brain injury
- Post-cardiac arrest myocardial dysfunction
- Systemic ischaemia/reperfusion response
- Persisting precipitating pathology

The severity of the post-cardiac arrest syndrome varies with the duration and cause of cardiac arrest; it may be absent if the

ABC of Resuscitation, Sixth Edition. Edited by Jasmeet Soar, Gavin D. Perkins and Jerry Nolan.
© 2013 John Wiley & Sons, Ltd. Published 2013 by John Wiley & Sons, Ltd.

cardiac arrest is brief. Post-cardiac arrest brain injury manifests as coma, seizures, myoclonus, varying degrees of neurological dysfunction and brain death. Post-cardiac arrest brain injury may be exacerbated by microcirculatory failure, impaired autoregulation, hypercarbia, hypoxaemia and hyperoxaemia, pyrexia, hyperglycaemia and seizures. Significant myocardial dysfunction is common after cardiac arrest but typically recovers by 2–3 days. The whole body ischaemia/reperfusion that occurs with resuscitation from cardiac arrest activates immunological and coagulation pathways contributing to multiple organ failure and increasing the risk of infection. Thus, the post-cardiac arrest syndrome has many features in common with sepsis, including intravascular volume depletion and vasodilation. About 60% of patients initially comatose after out-of-hospital cardiac arrest (OHCA) will develop pneumonia.

Optimising organ function

Airway and breathing

Patients who have had brief period of cardiac arrest may recover consciousness, maintain their airway safely and breathe adequately without the need for tracheal intubation. Patients remaining comatose and those with inadequate breathing will need support with mechanical ventilation via a tracheal tube.

Several animal studies indicate that hyperoxaemia causes oxidative stress and harms post-ischaemic neurones. Although the clinical data supporting this phenomenon are inconsistent, current recommendations are to titrate the inspired oxygen concentration to maintain the arterial blood oxygen saturation in the range of 94–98% as soon as arterial blood oxygen saturation can be monitored reliably (by blood gas analysis and/or pulse oximetry (SpO_2)). Adjust ventilation to achieve normocarbia and monitor this using the end-tidal CO_2 with waveform capnography and arterial blood gas values.

Circulation

Coronary artery disease is the most common cause of OHCA and many of these arrests will be associated with ST-segment elevation myocardial infarction (STEMI) for which early reperfusion therapy is required. Reperfusion can be achieved with primary percutaneous coronary intervention (PCI), fibrinolysis or both. Primary PCI is the preferred treatment if a first medical contact-to-balloon time of <90 min can be achieved because it is much more likely to establish full reperfusion than using fibrinolytic therapy. The early post-resuscitation 12-lead electrocardiogram (ECG) is less reliable for predicting acute coronary occlusion than it is in those who have not had a cardiac arrest. Recent evidence suggests that about 25% of patients with no obvious extra cardiac cause for their cardiac arrest but who do not have evidence of STEMI on their initial 12-lead ECG, will have a coronary lesion on angiography that is amenable to stenting. The trend is to consider immediate coronary artery angiography in all OHCA patients with no obvious non-cardiac cause of arrest.

Post-cardiac arrest myocardial dysfunction causes haemodynamic instability, which manifests as hypotension, a low cardiac output and arrhythmias. Early echocardiography will enable the extent of myocardial dysfunction to be quantified. In the ICU, an arterial line for continuous blood pressure monitoring is essential. Treatment with fluid, inotropes and vasopressors may be guided by blood pressure, heart rate, urine output, and rate of plasma lactate clearance and central venous oxygen saturations. Non-invasive cardiac output monitors may help to guide treatment. If treatment with fluid resuscitation and vasoactive drugs is insufficient to support the circulation, consider insertion of an intra-aortic balloon pump. In the absence of definitive data supporting a specific goal for blood pressure, target the mean arterial blood pressure to achieve an adequate urine output ($1\,ml\,kg^{-1}\,h^{-1}$) and normal or decreasing plasma lactate values, taking into consideration the patient's normal blood pressure, the cause of the arrest and the severity of any myocardial dysfunction.

Brain

In patients surviving to ICU admission but subsequently dying in hospital, brain injury is the cause of death in 68% after OHCA and in 23% after in-hospital cardiac arrest.

Cerebral perfusion

Immediately after ROSC, there is a period of cerebral hyperaemia. After asphyxial cardiac arrest, brain oedema may occur transiently after ROSC but it is associated only rarely with clinically relevant increases in intracranial pressure. Autoregulation of cerebral blood flow is impaired after cardiac arrest; thus, cerebral perfusion varies with cerebral perfusion pressure instead of being linked to neuronal activity. Maintain mean arterial pressure near the patient's normal level.

Sedation

There are no data to support a defined period of ventilation, sedation and neuromuscular blockade after cardiac arrest; however, patients need to be well sedated during treatment with therapeutic hypothermia, and the duration of sedation and ventilation is influenced by this treatment. Sedation is achieved typically with a combination of opioids and hypnotics. Short-acting drugs (e.g. propofol, alfentanil, remifentanil) will enable earlier neurological assessment. Adequate sedation will reduce oxygen consumption. During hypothermia, optimal sedation can reduce or prevent shivering, which enables the target temperature to be achieved

more rapidly. Mild hypothermia reduces clearance of many drugs by at least a third and may make later prognostication unreliable.

Control of seizures

Seizures or myoclonus or both occur in 10–40% of those who remain comatose after cardiac arrest. Although patients with seizures have four times the mortality rate of comatose patients without seizures, good neurological recovery has been documented in 17% of those with seizures. Seizures increase cerebral metabolism by up to threefold and may cause cerebral injury: treat with benzodiazepines, phenytoin, sodium valproate, propofol, or a barbiturate. Myoclonus can be particularly difficult to treat; phenytoin is often ineffective and may be best avoided. Clonazepam is the most effective antimyoclonic drug, but sodium valproate, levetiracetam and propofol can also be effective.

Glucose control

There is a strong association between high blood glucose after resuscitation from cardiac arrest and poor neurological outcome. However, severe hypoglycaemia is associated with increased mortality in critically ill patients and comatose patients are at particular risk from unrecognised hypoglycaemia. Based on the available data and expert consensus, following ROSC, blood glucose should be maintained at $\leq 10\,mmol\,l^{-1}$. Avoid hypoglycaemia ($<4.0\,mmol\,l^{-1}$).

Targeted temperature management

Pyrexia is common in the first 48 h after cardiac arrest and is associated with poor outcome; therefore, treat any hyperthermia occurring after cardiac arrest with antipyretics or active cooling.

Mild hypothermia is neuroprotective and improves outcome after a period of global cerebral hypoxia-ischaemia. Cooling suppresses many of the pathways leading to delayed cell death, including apoptosis (programmed cell death). Hypothermia decreases the cerebral metabolic rate for oxygen by about 6% for each $1\,^{\circ}C$ reduction in temperature and this may reduce the release of excitatory amino acids and free radicals.

Which post-cardiac arrest patients should be cooled?

All studies of post-cardiac-arrest therapeutic hypothermia have included only patients in coma. There is good evidence supporting the use of induced hypothermia in comatose survivors of OHCA caused by VF. Two randomised trials demonstrated improved neurological outcome at hospital discharge or at 6 months in comatose patients after out-of-hospital VF cardiac arrest. Cooling was initiated within minutes to hours after ROSC and a temperature range of 32–$34\,^{\circ}C$ was maintained for 12–24 h. The evidence supporting the use of hypothermia after cardiac arrest from non-shockable rhythms and after in-hospital cardiac arrest is much weaker and based only on non-randomised observational studies.

How to cool

The practical application of therapeutic hypothermia comprises induction, maintenance and rewarming. Earlier cooling after ROSC probably produces better outcome. External and/or internal cooling techniques can be used to initiate cooling. An infusion of 30 ml kg^{-1} of 4 °C 0.9% sodium chloride or Hartmann's solution decreases core temperature by approximately 1.5 °C and this technique can be used to initiate cooling pre-hospital. Other methods of inducing and/or maintaining hypothermia are listed in Box 8.2.

Box 8.2 Methods for inducing and maintaining hypothermia

- Simple ice packs and/or wet towels (inexpensive but may be more time consuming for nursing staff, may result in greater temperature fluctuations, and do not enable controlled rewarming)
- Ice-cold fluids alone cannot be used to maintain hypothermia, but even the addition of simple ice packs may control the temperature adequately
- Cooling blankets or pads (Figure 8.1)
- Water or air circulating blankets
- Water circulating gel-coated pads
- Intravascular heat exchanger, placed usually in the femoral or subclavian veins (Figure 8.2)
- Intranasal cooling
- Cardiopulmonary bypass

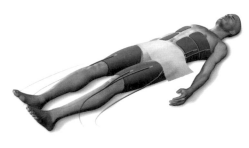

(a)

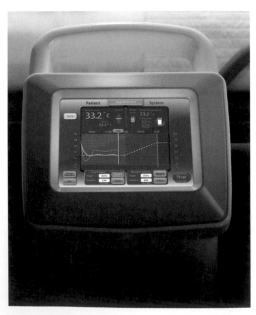

(b)

Figure 8.1 (a) and (b) Circulating water external temperature control system with feedback control. Images from http://www.medivance.com/AS5000Photos. © 2012 C. R. Bard, Inc. Used with permission. Arctic Sun Temperature Management® and ArcticGel™ Pad are trademarks and/or registered reademarks of C. R. Bard, Inc.

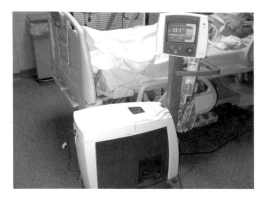

Figure 8.2 Intravascular temperature control system.

In most cases, it is easy to cool patients initially after ROSC because the temperature usually decreases spontaneously within this first hour. Shivering is prevented with sedation and bolus doses of neuromuscular blocker, as required. Magnesium sulphate (e.g. 5 g infused over 5 h) will reduce the shivering threshold.

Maintenance of target temperature is best achieved with external or internal cooling devices that include continuous temperature feedback to achieve a set target temperature. The temperature is typically monitored from a thermistor placed in the bladder and/or oesophagus. There are no data indicating that any specific cooling technique increases survival when compared with any other cooling technique; however, internal devices enable more precise temperature control compared with external techniques. The temperature is maintained in the target range (32–34 °C) for 24 h followed by slow, controlled rewarming at 0.25–0.5 °C of warming per hour and strict avoidance of hyperthermia. Plasma electrolyte concentrations, effective intravascular volume and metabolic rate can change rapidly during rewarming, as they do during cooling.

Physiological effects and complications of hypothermia
The well-recognised physiological effects of hypothermia (Box 8.3) need to be managed carefully.

Box 8.3 Physiological effects and complications of mild hypothermia

- Shivering – increases metabolic and heat production, and reduces cooling rates
- Increased systemic vascular resistance, arrhythmias (usually bradycardia)
- Diuresis and electrolyte abnormalities such as hypophosphataemia, hypokalaemia, hypomagnesaemia and hypocalcaemia
- Decreased insulin sensitivity and insulin secretion causing hyperglycaemia
- Impaired coagulation and increased bleeding
- Impaired immune response and increased infection, especially pneumonia
- Increased serum amylase
- Clearance of sedative drugs and neuromuscular blockers reduced by up to 30% at a core temperature of 34 °C

Contraindications to hypothermia

Generally recognised contraindications to therapeutic hypothermia, but which are not applied universally, include: severe systemic infection, established multiple organ failure and pre-existing medical coagulopathy (fibrinolytic therapy is not a contraindication to therapeutic hypothermia).

Prognostication

Predicting the eventual outcome of those remaining comatose after initial resuscitation from cardiac arrest is challenging. Clinicians would not wish to withdraw treatment if there is a realistic chance that the patient could eventually make a good neurological recovery; however, relentless treatment of a patient who is not going to make a good recovery is potentially distressing for relatives and is expensive. Three days after cardiac arrest and in the absence of sedation, a motor response to pain comprising extension or nothing, or fixed dilated pupils, or absent corneal reflexes, all used to be regarded as reliable indications of a poor outcome. However, these well-established guidelines were based on data generated before the widespread implementation of hypothermia. The use of hypothermia, and the increased sedation often given with this therapy, can delay recovery of motor reaction for 5–6 days after cardiac arrest. Based on recent data, following use of therapeutic hypothermia, reliable prognostication cannot be achieved until 3 days after return to normothermia. The most reliable approach to prognostication is multimodal: the presence of at least two independent predictors out of four (incomplete recovery of brainstem reflexes, myoclonus, an unreactive electroencephalogram (EEG), and absent cortical somatosensory evoked potentials (SSEPs)) reliably indicate a poor outcome. The major limitation to these recommendations is that in most hospitals it is often difficult or impossible to access some of these more sophisticated neurological investigations.

Organ donation

Up to 16% of patients who achieve sustained ROSC after cardiac arrest develop clinical brain death and can be considered for organ donation. Transplant outcomes from the use of these organs are similar to those achieved with organs from other brain-dead donors.

Further reading

Deakin CD, Morrison LJ, Morley PT, *et al*. Part 8: Advanced life support: 2010 International Consensus on Cardiopulmonary Resuscitation and Emergency Cardiovascular Care Science with Treatment Recommendations. *Resuscitation* 2010;**81**(Suppl 1):e93-e174.

Deakin CD, Nolan JP, Soar J, *et al*. European Resuscitation Council Guidelines for Resuscitation 2010 Section 4. Adult advanced life support. *Resuscitation* 2010;**81**:1305–52.

Nolan JP, Neumar RW, Adrie C, *et al*. Post-cardiac arrest syndrome: epidemiology, pathophysiology, treatment, and prognostication. A Scientific Statement from the International Liaison Committee on Resuscitation; the American Heart Association Emergency Cardiovascular Care Committee; the Council on Cardiovascular Surgery and Anesthesia; the Council on Cardiopulmonary, Perioperative, and Critical Care; the Council on Clinical Cardiology; the Council on Stroke. *Resuscitation* 2008;**79**:350–79.

Nolan JP, Soar J. Postresuscitation care: entering a new era. *Curr Opin Crit Care* 2010;**16**:216–22.

Rossetti AO, Oddo M, Logroscino G, Kaplan PW. Prognostication after cardiac arrest and hypothermia: a prospective study. *Ann Neurol* 2010;**67**:301–7.

CHAPTER 9

Paediatric Resuscitation

Ian K. Maconochie[1] and Robert Bingham[2]

[1]St. Mary's Hospital, London, UK
[2]Great Ormond Street Children's Hospital, London, UK

OVERVIEW

- Early detection and treatment of the deteriorating child can prevent cardiac arrest
- High-quality chest compressions with ventilations are important to improve outcomes
- Once CPR has started, minimise interruptions in chest compressions for other interventions such as defibrillation and tracheal intubation

Introduction

Paediatric cardiorespiratory arrest is often caused by hypoxia, as the body has limited compensatory mechanisms to deal with severe illness or injury. Ventricular fibrillation or pulseless ventricular tachycardia is uncommon in children compared to adults, as primary heart disease occurs infrequently. Pronounced hypoxia arising from progressive illness (or the effects of injury) causes myocardial dysfunction, leading to profound bradycardia, which can degenerate to asystole or pulseless electrical activity (PEA). Other vital organs also suffer from severe hypoxia. Both asystole and PEA have poor outcomes.

The body's initial response is to adapt by altering respiratory or circulatory parameters, depending on the underlying condition, for example respiratory disease such as asthma will lead to changes in respiratory parameters which may lead in turn to changes in the circulation. If the body is unable to deal with the illness/injury, the compensatory changes may not be sustainable, leading to decompensated respiratory and/or circulatory failure (Figure 9.1).

These may combine as the body's physiological responses further decline, leading to cardiorespiratory failure and, if unchecked, cardiorespiratory arrest.

Morbidity and mortality remain high if cardiorespiratory arrest occurs, as the profound hypoxia leads to multi-organ failure in many cases. For cardiorespiratory arrests that occur out of hospital, survival is between 6 and 12%, with fewer than 5% having no neurological consequences. In hospital, 27% of cardiac arrest patients survive to discharge, and of those having a respiratory

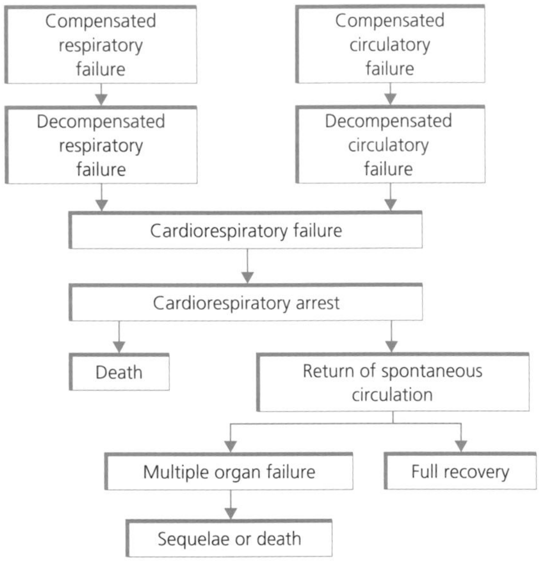

Figure 9.1 The sequence of events in the seriously ill/injured child who deteriorates over time (with permission from Resuscitation Council UK).

arrest where cardiac output is still maintained, more than 70% have good long-term outcomes.

These figures highlight the importance of recognising the symptoms and signs of the body's physiological responses to illness or injury as early as possible, as interventions can reverse the deterioration to cardiorespiratory arrest.

Paediatric basic life support

Treatment should follow the sequence – **A**irway, **B**reathing **C**irculation. There are differences from adult practice as the most common cause of cardiorespiratory arrest is hypoxia, hence the need to deliver oxygen from the outset. The key steps are outlined in the paediatric basic life support algorithm (Figure 9.2). This guidance is aimed predominantly at those with a duty to respond to paediatric emergencies. For those with no paediatric training or who have forgotten, or are unsure of, the correct paediatric sequence; it is perfectly acceptable, and far better than doing nothing, to use the adult sequence (see Chapter 4).

ABC of Resuscitation, Sixth Edition. Edited by Jasmeet Soar, Gavin D. Perkins and Jerry Nolan.
© 2013 John Wiley & Sons, Ltd. Published 2013 by John Wiley & Sons, Ltd.

Paediatric Basic Life Support
(Healthcare professionals with a duty to respond)

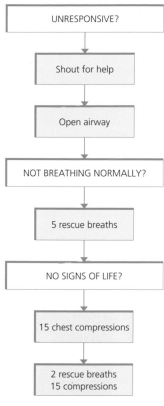

```
┌─────────────────────────┐
│      UNRESPONSIVE?       │
└─────────────────────────┘
            │
            ▼
┌─────────────────────────┐
│      Shout for help      │
└─────────────────────────┘
            │
            ▼
┌─────────────────────────┐
│       Open airway        │
└─────────────────────────┘
            │
            ▼
┌─────────────────────────┐
│  NOT BREATHING NORMALLY? │
└─────────────────────────┘
            │
            ▼
┌─────────────────────────┐
│     5 rescue breaths     │
└─────────────────────────┘
            │
            ▼
┌─────────────────────────┐
│     NO SIGNS OF LIFE?    │
└─────────────────────────┘
            │
            ▼
┌─────────────────────────┐
│   15 chest compressions  │
└─────────────────────────┘
            │
            ▼
┌─────────────────────────┐
│     2 rescue breaths     │
│     15 compressions      │
└─────────────────────────┘
```

Call resuscitation team

Figure 9.2 Paediatric basic life support algorithm. Reproduced with the kind permission of the Resuscitation Council (UK).

Unresponsive?

After confirming there are no dangers, the first stage is to confirm unresponsiveness. This may be done by gentle stimulation of the infant/young children, saying 'Are you alright?' and observing for any response, such as movement or breathing.

Should the child be unconscious but have a regular breathing pattern, it may be best to place them in the recovery position if there are no signs of trauma.

Shout for help

If there is no response, then shout for help. If someone comes to your aid, ask them to alert emergency services, telling them to give: the location of the child, the child's approximate age and that basic life support is being given. Tell the person to return to you after they have done this.

Open the airway

Open the airway by performing a head tilt, chin lift technique (Figure 9.3). Look inside the mouth to see if there is any foreign body that can be directly extracted. Look for chest wall movement, listen for any spontaneous breathing and feel if there is expired air on your cheek for no more than 10 seconds. If normal breathing is absent, you will have to deliver 5 rescue breaths.

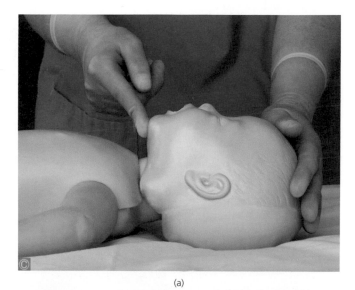

(a)

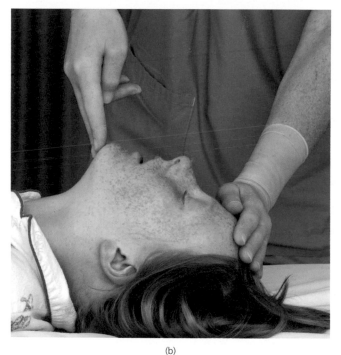

(b)

Figure 9.3 Head tilt and chin lift in (a) an infant and (b) a child. Photograph reproduced with kind permission by Michael Scott and the Resuscitation Council (UK).

Irregular gasping (agonal) breaths are not normal and rescue breathing should be performed.

Five rescue breaths

To deliver rescue breaths, put your mouth over the child's, pinch the nose to occlude it and blow slowly (over about 1 to 1.5 s) in order to make the child's chest rise as for a normal breath. For an infant, it may be easier to put your mouth on their face so that both the mouth and nose is covered (Figure 9.4). Look for chest wall movement to ensure the chest gently rises and falls with each breath you deliver. If the chest wall does not move, re-position the head,

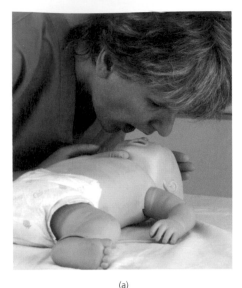
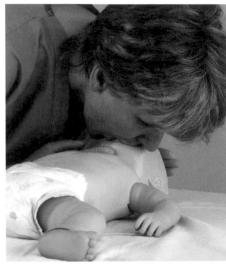

Figure 9.4 (a) and (b) Mouth to nose ventilation in an infant. Photograph reproduced with kind permission by Michael Scott and the Resuscitation Council (UK).

(a)

(b)

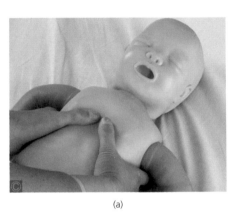
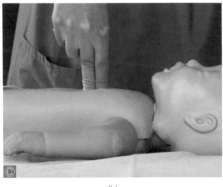
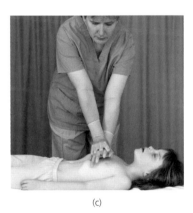

(a)

(b)

(c)

Figure 9.5 Chest compression in an infant with (a) a two-thumb encircling technique, (b) a two-finger technique and (c) in a child with a two-handed technique. Photograph reproduced with kind permission by Michael Scott and the Resuscitation Council (UK).

before performing the next breath in the sequence, as the airway may not be open.

No signs of life?

Then assess for signs of a circulation. This should take no more than 10 s. Look for signs of life (e.g. movement or regular breathing) and feel for a pulse. In an infant, feel for a pulse in a brachial artery, and in the older child, the carotid artery. In both age groups, a femoral artery may be palpated. Palpation of the pulse cannot be the sole determinant of the need for chest compressions.

If you are sure there are signs of life or a pulse of >60 beats min^{-1}, continue giving breaths until the child/infant starts breathing regularly, when he should be turned into the lateral recovery position.

Chest compressions

If there are no signs of life or a pulse of >60 min^{-1}, **or you are not sure**, the next stage is to deliver 15 chest compressions. In the infant, if there are two rescuers, the infant's thorax may be

encircled by the rescuer's hands, and the two thumbs used to deliver compressions, allowing the other rescuer to give the rescue breaths. A single rescuer may find it easier to use 2 fingers of one hand. In children, one or two hands should be used to achieve the correct compression depth (Figure 9.5).

For all infants and children, compression should be over the lower half of the sternum to a depth of at least one-third of the anterior posterior diameter of the chest (approximately 4 cm in an infant and 5 cm in an older child). The rate of compression should be at least 100 but not >120 min^{-1}. About the same amount of time should be spent in the compressed phase as in the released phase, with complete release of pressure each time. Physical damage following chest compressions in children is relatively uncommon. It is therefore reasonable to advise, 'Don't be afraid to push too hard'.

Two breaths followed by 15 chest compressions

Open the airway and deliver a further 2 breaths, followed by 15 chest compressions as previously. CPR should continue using a 2:15 ratio of breaths to chest compressions.

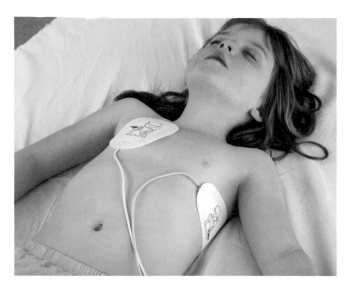

Figure 9.6 Defibrillator pad position. Photograph reproduced with kind permission by Michael Scott and the Resuscitation Council (UK).

Deliver 1 minute of basic life support before going for help, if there is no one to go for you. It may be possible to take the infant or small child with you. If you know help is coming, continue with the sequence of 2 breaths to 15 chest compressions.

When to stop

Resuscitation should continue until expert help arrives and can take over, or if there are signs of life (return of consciousness, normal breathing, cough, purposeful movement or pulse of > 60 beats min^{-1}) or if you become exhausted.

Automated external defibrillator (AED) use in children

A standard 'adult' AED with adult pads can be used in children. Ideally, an AED with an attenuating device should be used in children between 1 and 8 years old (<25 kg). In addition, if there is any possibility that an AED may need to be used in children, the purchaser should check that the performance of the particular model has been tested in paediatric arrhythmias. Shockable cardiac arrest rhythms are uncommon in infants (<1 year old). There are case reports of the successful use of AEDs in this age group and the risk:benefit ratio favours the use of an AED (ideally with an attenuator) if a manual defibrillator is not available.

AED pads should be placed below the right clavicle and at the cardiac apex in the mid-axillary line (Figure 9.6). If the pads are too large or only adult pads are available, the pads should be placed anterior-posterior on the chest and back to avoid contact between the two pads. The AED should be switched on and the audio-visual prompts followed.

Paediatric advanced life support

Paediatric advanced life support is critically dependant on the delivery of high-quality basic life support. The management follows the same ABC sequence, used for the treatment of any ill or injured child. The key steps are outlined in the paediatric advanced life support algorithm (Figure 9.7). Table 9.1 summarises key information required for paediatric advanced life support.

Step 1
Continue with high-quality basic life support.

As soon as it is available, use bag-mask ventilation with high-flow oxygen. Airway adjuncts such as oral airways may be placed and tracheal intubation should be considered if there are clinicians present who are trained in this procedure. Expired carbon dioxide monitoring should be employed, if possible. When the trachea is intubated, the ventilation rate should be 10–12 breaths min^{-1} together with continuous chest compressions at 100–120 min^{-1}.

Step 2
Place monitors to determine if there is a 'shockable rhythm' or 'non-shockable rhythm' and assess for signs of life (cough, movement or a regular breathing).

The monitor can be a defibrillator or a separate ECG monitor.

Shockable rhythm (ventricular fibrillation (VF) or pulseless ventricular tachycardia (VT)) should be defibrillated as soon as possible.

Step 3
For a non-shockable rhythm (asystole, profound bradycardia and pulseless electrical activity)

Maintain high-quality CPR, secure vascular access then give adrenaline 10 microgram kg^{-1} bodyweight. Intraosseous (IO) access is preferred in CPR if intravenous access is not already present.

Continue CPR for 2 min, then stop briefly to check the rhythm on the monitor.

Repeat the adrenaline dose every 3–5 min, i.e. every other loop.

Look for the reversible causes – mnemonic: 4Hs and the 4Ts:

- Hypoxia
- Hypovolaemia
- Hypoalaemia/hyperkalaemia/metabolic
- Hypothermia
- Tension pneumothorax
- Toxins
- Tamponade – cardiac
- Thromboembolism

For a shockable rhythm (VF or pulseless VT)
a. Maintain high-quality CPR until a defibrillator is ready
b. Pads are placed on the chest and the defibrillator is charged whilst chest compression continues. After ensuring that no one is in contact with the patient, deliver a shock of 4 J kg^{-1} bodyweight
c. Immediately resume CPR, without checking the monitor

d. Consider reversible causes – 4Hs and 4Ts (as earlier)
e. After 2 min, stop briefly to check the monitor – if no change, then repeat shock at 4 J kg^{-1}
f. Immediately resume CPR
g. After 2 min, stop CPR and check the monitor – if no change, repeat shock at same energy
h. After resuming CPR, give adrenaline 10 microgram kg^{-1} and amiodarone 5 mg kg^{-1} bodyweight

Repeat adrenaline at the same dose every 3–5 minute until there is a return to spontaneous circulation. The same dosage of amiodarone may be given, after the fifth shock if the patient is still in a shockable rhythm.

Every 2 minutes, the monitor should be checked.

Should it show VF/pulseless VT, continue with the shockable sequence.

If the monitor shows asystole, change to the non-shockable sequence.

If there is organised electrical activity, check for signs of life and a pulse:

- If there are no signs of life or the pulse is less than 60 beats min^{-1}, continue CPR by the non-shockable sequence
- If there are signs of life or a pulse >60 beats min^{-1}, start post-resuscitation care.

Parental presence

Many parents wish to be present during a resuscitation attempt so they can see that everything possible is being done for their child. This can be comforting to parents or carers and can help the bereavement process if resuscitation is unsuccessful. A dedicated staff member should stay with the parents and explain the

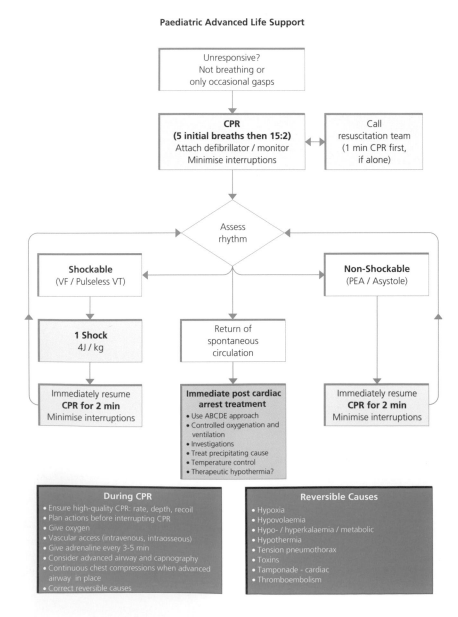

Figure 9.7 Paediatric advanced life support algorithm. Reproduced with the kind permission of the Resuscitation Council (UK).

Table 9.1 Paediatric Emergency Treatment Chart.

		ADRENALINE	FLUID BOLUS	GLUCOSE	SODIUM BICARBONATE		TRACHEAL TUBE UNCUFFED	TRACHEAL TUBE CUFFED	DEFIBRILLATION
	STRENGTH DOSE	1:10,000 10 microgram kg^{-1}	0.9% Saline 20 ml kg^{-1}	10% 2 ml kg^{-1}	4.2% 1 mmol kg^{-1}	8.4%			4 Joules kg^{-1}
	ROUTE	IV, IO	IV, IO	IV, IO	IV, IO, UVC	IV, IO			Trans-thoracic
	NOTES		Consider warmed fluids	For known hypoglycaemia				Monitor cuff pressure	Monophasic or biphasic
AGE	WEIGHT kg	ml	ml	Recheck glucose after dose ml	ml	ml	ID mm	ID mm	Manual
<1 month	3.5	0.35	70	7	7	-	3.0	-	20
1 month	4	0.4	80	8	8	-	3.0–3.5	3.0	20
3 months	5	0.5	100	10	10	-	3.5	3.0	20
6 months	7	0.7	140	14	-	7	3.5	3.0	30
1 year	10	1.0	200	20	-	10	4.0	3.5	40
2 years	12	1.2	240	24	-	12	4.5	4.0	50
3 years	14	1.4	280	28	-	14	4.5–5.0	4.0–4.5	60
4 years	16	1.6	320	32	-	16	5.0	4.5	60
5 years	18	1.8	360	36	-	18	5.0–5.5	4.5–5.0	70
6 years	20	2.0	400	40	-	20	5.5	5.0	80
7 years	23	2.3	460	46	-	23	5.5–6.0	5.0–5.5	90
8 years	26	2.6	520	52	-	26	-	6.0–6.5	100
10 years	30	3.0	600	60	-	30	-	7.0	120
12 years	38	3.8	760	76	-	38	-	7–7.5	150
Adolescent	>40 kg	10	1000	80	-	50	-	7–8	As for adults

Cardioversion	Synchronised Shock – 0.5–1.0 Joules kg^{-1} escalating to 2.0 Joules kg^{-1} if unsuccessful.
Amiodarone	5 mg kg^{-1} IV or IO bolus in arrest (0.1 ml kg^{-1} of 150 mg in 3 ml) after 3rd and 5th shocks. Flush line with 0.9% saline or 5% glucose.
Atropine	20 microgram kg^{-1}, minimum dose 100 microgram, maximum dose 600 microgram.
Calcium chloride 10%	0.2 ml kg^{-1} for hypocalcaemia / hyperkalaemia.
Lorazepam	100 microgram kg^{-1} IV or IO for treatment of seizures. Can be repeated after 10 minutes. Maximum single dose 4 mg.
Naloxone	Resuscitation dose for full reversal 100 microgram kg^{-1}. For partial reversal of opiate analgesia 10 microgram kg^{-1} boluses, titrated to effect.
Anaphylaxis	Adrenaline 1:1000 intramuscularly (<6 yrs 150 microgram [0.15 ml], 6–12 yrs 300 microgram [0.3 ml], >12 yrs 500 microgram [0.5 ml]) can be repeated after five minutes. OR titrate boluses of 1 microgram kg^{-1} IV ONLY if familiar with giving IV adrenaline.

Weights averaged on lean body mass from 50th centile weights for males and females. Drug doses based on Resuscitation Council (UK) Guidelines 2010 recommendations. Recommendations for tracheal tubes are based on full term neonates. For newborns glucose at 2.5 ml kg^{-1} is recommended.

process in an empathetic and sympathetic manner. Physical contact with the child should be allowed. If parental presence impedes the resuscitation attempt, the parents should be gently asked to leave.

Choking

Recognition of choking

Usually spontaneous coughing will expel any foreign body from the airway. If coughing is absent or ineffective, back blows, chest thrusts and abdominal thrusts can expel foreign bodies from the airway by increasing intrathoracic pressure. More than one technique is often needed to relieve the obstruction. If one is unsuccessful, try the others in rotation until the object is cleared.

Choking causes sudden onset of respiratory distress associated with coughing, gagging, or stridor. Other causes of airway obstruction, such as laryngitis or epiglottitis can cause similar signs. Table 9.2 lists signs and symptoms to help diagnose choking.

Table 9.2 Signs and symptoms of choking in children.

General signs of choking	Witnessed episode Coughing or choking Sudden onset No other signs of illness Recent history of playing with or eating small objects
Ineffective cough	Unable to vocalise Quiet or silent cough Unable to breathe Cyanosis Decreasing level of consciousness
Effective cough	Crying or verbal response to questions Loud cough Able to take a breath before coughing Fully responsive

Treatment of choking in children

The treatment of choking in children in summarised in the paediatric choking treatment algorithm (Figure 9.8).

Paediatric Choking Treatment Algorithm

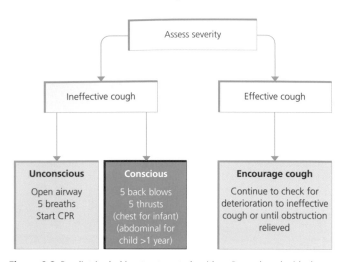

Figure 9.8 Paediatric choking treatment algorithm. Reproduced with the kind permission of the Resuscitation Council (UK).

Conscious child with choking

- For back-blows support infant in a head-downwards, prone position, to enable gravity to assist removal of the foreign body. A small child may be placed across the rescuer's lap as with an infant
- Give back blows with the heel of one hand in the middle of the back between the shoulder blades – the aim is to relieve the obstruction with each blow rather than give all five
- Chest thrusts are similar to chest compressions, but sharper in nature and delivered at a slower rate
- Abdominal thrusts should not be used in children under 1 year. For abdominal thrusts, stand or kneel behind the child. Clench your fist and place it between the umbilicus and xiphisternum. Grasp this hand with your other hand and pull sharply inwards and upwards

- If the object has not been expelled and the victim is still conscious, continue the sequence of back blows and chest (for infant) or abdominal (for children) thrusts
- If the object is expelled, assess the child's clinical condition. Part of the object can remain in the respiratory tract and cause complications. If there is any doubt, seek medical assistance

Unconscious child with choking

- If the child is, or becomes, unconscious, place on a firm, flat surface, and ensure help is coming
- Open the mouth and look for any obvious object – if an object is seen, remove with a single finger sweep. Do not use blind or repeated finger sweeps as they can push the object further down the airway and worsen the situation
- Open the airway and attempt five rescue breaths as during basic life support – if a breath does not make the chest rise, reposition the head before making the next attempt
- Attempt five rescue breaths and if there is no response, proceed immediately to chest compression regardless of whether the breaths are successful
- Give 1 min of CPR before getting help if help has not already been summoned by someone else
- When giving rescue breaths, look for an object in the airway and remove if seen
- Continue CPR unless the child regains consciousness and is breathing effectively or until expert help arrives

Further reading

Biarent D, Bingham R, Eich C, *et al.* European Resuscitation Council Guidelines for Resuscitation 2010 Section 6. Paediatric life support. *Resuscitation* 2010;**81**:1364–88.

de Caen AR, Kleinman ME, Chameides L, *et al.* Part 10: Paediatric basic and advanced life support: 2010 International Consensus on Cardiopulmonary Resuscitation and Emergency Cardiovascular Care Science with Treatment Recommendations. *Resuscitation* 2010;**81**(Supp 1):e213–59.

CHAPTER 10

Resuscitation at Birth

Jonathan Wyllie[1] and Sean Ainsworth[2]

[1] The James Cook University Hospital, Middlesborough, UK
[2] Victoria Hospital, Kirkcaldy, UK

OVERVIEW

- Although delivery of an apparently lifeless baby is a rare event, systems must be in place to ensure prompt and effective initiation of life support
- Resuscitation equipment should be readily available and must include facilities for temperature control to keep the newborn warm
- Initial steps during delivery comprise keeping the baby warm and assessing respiration, heart rate, colour and tone
- If resuscitation is required following the Airway, Breathing Circulation sequence
- When possible, use pulse oximetry to monitor oxygen saturations and heart rate. Avoid hyperoxia in the premature infant

---

Introduction

Most babies make the transition to extrauterine life without assistance and breathe effectively within 90 s of birth. A small number need assistance with that transition and require airway management and sometimes establishment of breathing. The need for both ventilation and chest compressions in an apparently lifeless baby is a rare event affecting less than 0.1% of births. However, every newborn baby should be assessed at birth by someone who is trained in basic newborn resuscitation.

Babies considered to be at increased risk (Box 10.1) should be delivered in a unit with full newborn life support facilities. Delivery units should have guidelines to ensure appropriately trained professionals are available for such deliveries. These guidelines might entail attendance at 25% of all births, although most babies will not require any assistance. Even with such guidelines, help may still be unexpectedly required in a further 1.5% of births. This unpredictable need for resuscitation highlights the need for recognised newborn resuscitation courses (Box 10.2).

Equipment and temperature control

As the need for resuscitation cannot always be predicted, it is useful to plan for such an eventuality. Equipment that may be used to

---

Box 10.1 **Factors that increase the risk of a newborn requiring resuscitation**

Maternal

- Severe pregnancy-induced hypertension
- Diabetes mellitus
- Heavy sedation
- Severe maternal illness

Delivery

- Evidence of fetal compromise
- Abnormal presentation
- Prolapsed umbilical cord
- Antepartum haemorrhage
- Thick or old particulate meconium
- High instrumental delivery
- Class 1 caesarean section

Fetal

- Multiple pregnancy
- Prematurity (<34 weeks)
- Post-maturity (>42 weeks)
- In utero growth restriction
- Rhesus isoimmunisation
- Polyhydramnios and oligohydramnios
- Severe fetal abnormality

Box 10.2 **Recognised newborn resuscitation courses and website details**

Newborn Life Support course, Resuscitation Council (UK). Website: http://www.resus.org.uk/pages/nlsinfo.htm
European Resuscitation Council. Website: https://www.erc.edu/index.php/mainpage/en/
Neonatal Resuscitation Program™, American Academy of Pediatrics. Website: http://www2.aap.org/nrp/default.html

---

resuscitate a newborn baby is listed in Box 10.3. This is not an essential or exhaustive list and will vary between institutions. An appropriately trained person needs, as a minimum, a flat surface, warmth and a way to deliver air or oxygen at a controlled pressure. In delivery units, a resuscitaire fulfils these latter requirements. Current recommendations are to commence resuscitation with air

ABC of Resuscitation, Sixth Edition. Edited by Jasmeet Soar, Gavin D. Perkins and Jerry Nolan.
© 2013 John Wiley & Sons, Ltd. Published 2013 by John Wiley & Sons, Ltd.

and most modern resuscitaires have air–oxygen blenders which provide oxygen concentrations of 21–100%. It is the responsibility of all professionals to be fully conversant with the equipment available in their place of work.

Box 10.3 **Equipment for newborn resuscitation**

- A flat surface (resuscitaire in hospital)
- A source of warmth and dry towels
- A plastic wrap or bag and radiant heater for preterm babies
- A suction system with at least 12 FG catheters
- Face masks
- Self-inflating bag (500 ml) with pressure release valve or pressure-limiting device
- Source of air and/or oxygen
- Oropharyngeal airways
- Laryngoscopes with straight size 0 and 1 blades
- Nasogastric tubes
- Umbilical cord clamp
- Scissors
- Tracheal tubes 2.5–4.0 mm diameter
- Tracheal tube stylet
- Umbilical catheterisation set
- Adhesive tape
- Disposable gloves
- Stethoscope and saturation monitor

Maintaining the baby's temperature with dry covers and a radiant heater is essential, as even in environments of 20–24 °C the core temperature of vulnerable babies may drop by 5 °C in as many minutes.

Procedure at delivery

If time allows, ensure that equipment is ready and, if appropriate, introduce yourself to the parents. There is usually no need to immediately clamp the cord, particularly if the baby seems well. Unless the baby is clearly in need of immediate resuscitation, cord clamping can be delayed for at least 1 min after the complete delivery of the baby. Keep the baby warm and assess whether any intervention is going to be needed. If the baby is thought to need assistance, then this takes precedence and the cord may need to be clamped in order to deliver that assistance. Aspirating the pharynx used to be common practice but this is almost always unnecessary and it may cause a delay in spontaneous respirations and bradycardia.

Keeping the baby warm

With a large surface area to weight ratio, babies can lose heat very quickly. Dry the baby off immediately and then wrap in a dry towel. Cold babies use more oxygen and are more likely to become hypoglycaemic and acidotic. Ideally, delivery should take place in a warm room, and an overhead heater should be switched on. Overall, however, drying effectively and wrapping the baby using a warm

dry towel is the most important factor in avoiding hypothermia. Ensure that the head is covered as this represents a significant part of the baby's surface area.

A more effective way to keep small and low gestation babies (less than 28 weeks gestation) warm in the delivery room is to place them immediately (i.e. without drying) into a polythene covering and under a radiant heat source.

Assessment of the newborn baby

Whilst the baby is kept warm, an initial assessment is made of respiration, heart rate, colour and tone. Unlike resuscitation at other ages, it is essential to assess fully in order that one can judge the success of interventions. This is most true of *heart rate* and *breathing*, which guide further resuscitative efforts and which are the focus of subsequent assessments. However, a baby who is white and shut down peripherally is more likely to be acidotic and a baby who is atonic is likely to be unconscious.

Resuscitation procedure

Most babies will start breathing within 10–20 s and establish spontaneous regular breathing sufficient to maintain the heart rate above 100 min^{-1} and improve colour within 90–180 s of birth. If apnoea or gasping persists after drying, intervention is required. Resuscitation should then follow the most recent standardised guidelines. These acknowledge that relatively few resuscitation interventions have been subject to randomised controlled trials. They are, however, based on as wide an examination of the evidence as possible. Resuscitation follows a standard Airway, Breathing, Circulation pathway, with the use of drugs in a tiny minority of cases (Figure 10.1).

Airway

The baby's head should be placed in the neutral position. The occiput of a newborn baby is large and often moulded; in the supine baby this causes the neck to flex and the airway to close. Over extension may also collapse the newborn baby's pharyngeal airway. A 2-cm thickness of towel under the neck and shoulders can help to maintain the neutral position. In an atonic baby, jaw thrust may well be required to bring the tongue forward and open the airway.

Meconium

Meconium-stained liquor (light green tinge) is relatively common and occurs in up to 10% of births. However, meconium aspiration is a rare event and usually happens before delivery. Suctioning the airway whilst the head is on the perineum is not of benefit and may delay resuscitation; this practice is, therefore, not recommended. If the baby is vigorous, no specific action (other than drying and wrapping) is needed. If the baby has absent or inadequate respirations, a slow heart rate and/or hypotonia; inspect the oropharynx with a laryngoscope and aspirate any particulate meconium seen using a wide-bore catheter. If the baby is unresponsive and intubation is possible, aspirate the trachea using the tracheal tube as a suction catheter. If intubation cannot be achieved immediately, clear the

Newborn Life Support

Dry the baby Remove any wet towels and cover Start the clock or note the time	Birth	AT
Assess (tone), breathing and heart rate	30 sec	ALL
If gasping or not breathing: Open the airway Give 5 inflation breaths Consider SpO₂ monitoring	60 sec	STAGES
Re-assess If no increase in heart rate look for chest movement		ASK :

If chest not moving: Recheck head position Consider 2-person airway control and other airway manoeuvres Repeat inflation breaths Consider SpO₂ monitoring Look for a response	Acceptable pre-ductal SpO₂ 2 min 60% 3 min 70% 4 min 80% 5 min 85% 10 min 90%

If no increase in heart rate look for chest movement	DO
When the chest is moving: If heart rate is not detectable or slow (< 60 min⁻¹) Start chest compressions 3 compressions to each breath	YOU NEED
Reassess heart rate every 30 seconds If heart rate is not detectable or slow (<60 min⁻¹) consider venous access and drugs	HELP?

Figure 10.1 Standard resuscitation guidelines. Reproduced with the kind permission of the Resuscitation Council (UK).

oropharynx and start mask inflation. Over-zealous clearance of the airway can be detrimental, if the heart rate falls to < 60 min^{-1} stop airway clearance, give aeration breaths and start ventilation.

Tracheal intubation

Most babies can be resuscitated using a mask system. Swedish data suggests that if this is applied correctly, then only 1:500 babies actually *need* intubation. Tracheal intubation only remains gold standard airway management if it is performed perfectly. It is especially useful in prolonged resuscitations, preterm babies and meconium aspiration. It may be considered if mask ventilation has failed, although the most common reason for failure is poor positioning of the head with consequent failure to open the airway. A normal full-term newborn usually needs a 3.5-mm diameter tracheal tube, but other sizes (2.5, 3.0 and 4.0) should be available.

Tracheal tube placement must be assessed visually during intubation and in most cases will be confirmed by a rapid response in heart rate on ventilating. If in doubt, exhaled CO_2 detectors will correctly identify most correctly sited tubes in the presence of any cardiac output.

Breathing (aeration breaths and ventilation)

The purpose of the first five breaths delivered to term babies is to aerate the lungs. These should be sustained breaths (2–3 s) preferably using a continuous gas supply, a pressure-limiting device and a mask. If no such system is available, then a 500 ml self-inflating bag with a blow-off valve set at 30–40 cmH$_2$O can be used. This is especially useful in the absence of compressed air or oxygen. Use a mask big enough to cover the nose and mouth of the baby (Figure 10.2).

Adequate ventilation is usually indicated by either a rapidly increasing heart rate or a heart rate that is maintained at > 100 min^{-1}. Therefore, reassess the heart rate after the first five breaths. It is safe to assume that the chest has been successfully aerated if the heart rate responds. Ventilation should then be continued at a rate of 30–40 shorter breaths per minute until regular breathing is established. Where possible, start resuscitation using air. There is now good evidence for this in term babies and oxygen toxicity is a real concern with premature babies.

If the heart rate has not responded then check for chest movement rather than auscultation; in fluid-filled lungs breath sounds may be heard without lung inflation. Go back and check airway-opening manoeuvres and consider using a two-person approach to mask inflation (Figure 10.3). This has been shown to reduce mask leak and improve technique.

Circulation

If the heart rate remains slow or absent, despite adequate ventilation with chest movement for 30 s, then chest compressions should be

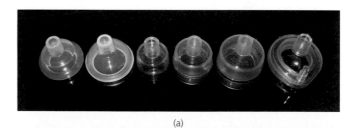

(a)

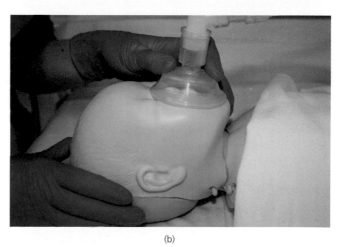

(b)

Figure 10.2 (a) Different types of masks for newborns. (b) Newborn baby manikin in neutral position with a well fitting mask. Thumb and forefinger applying mask with other three fingers supporting the jaw.

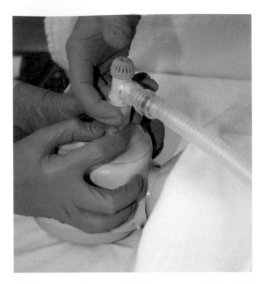

Figure 10.3 Two-person airway control. One person applying mask and delivering jaw thrust, the second delivering breaths.

started. Chest compressions aim to move oxygenated blood from the lungs to the heart and coronary arteries. The blood can only be oxygenated if the lungs are aerated. Cardiac compromise is always secondary to respiratory failure and can only be effectively treated if effective ventilation is occurring. The most efficient way of delivering chest compressions in the newborn is to encircle the chest with both hands, so that the fingers lie behind the baby and the thumbs are apposed on the sternum just below the inter-nipple line. Compress the chest briskly, *by one-third of its depth*. In newborn babies, current advice is to perform three compressions for each ventilation breath (3:1 ratio). Once the heart rate is above 60 min^{-1} and rising, chest compression should be discontinued. Maintain ventilation until effective breathing or mechanical ventilation is established.

Drugs

If the heart rate has not responded after adequate lung aeration, ventilation and cardiac compression, then drug therapy should be considered. The most common reason for the absence of a heart rate response is failure to achieve lung aeration and ventilation. Airway and breathing must be adequate before proceeding to drugs. Venous access will be required via an umbilical venous line because drugs should be given centrally. Adrenaline and bicarbonate are the most frequently used drugs, but dextrose and volume may also be required. Doses of drugs are given in Box 10.4.

Rarely, hypovolaemia may be present because of known or suspected blood loss (antepartum haemorrhage, placenta or vasa praevia, unclamped cord) or due to secondary to loss of vascular tone following asphyxia. Volume expansion, initially with 10 ml kg^{-1}, may be appropriate. An increase in heart rate is the usual sign of a response to any of these interventions.

Pre-term babies

The more immature a baby, the less likely it is to establish adequate respirations. A lack of surfactant, increased effort of respiration

---

Box 10.4 Drugs used in newborn resuscitation

Adrenaline (intravenous injection)
Initial dose:10 micogram/kg (0.1 ml of 1:10,000 solution)
Subsequent doses:10–30 microgram/kg (0.1–0.3 ml of 1:10,000 solution)
Comment:may be given via the tracheal tube at a dose of 50 microgram/kg (0.5 ml of 1:10,000 solution), but efficacy when administered via this route is not proven

Sodium bicarbonate (intravenous injection)
1 mmol/kg (2 ml kg^{-1} of 4.2% solution)

Dextrose (intravenous injection)
250 mg/kg (2.5 ml kg^{-1} of 10% dextrose)

Volume
10 ml/kg of 0.9% saline or other balanced salt solution

and a less developed chest musculature must be anticipated in babies born before 32 weeks. These babies may require assistance to establish aeration and ventilation and, in some cases, exogenous surfactant.

The lungs of preterm babies are much more susceptible to damage from over-distension than those of term babies. Resuscitation should start with lower inflation pressures of 20–25 cmH$_2$O, with the use of PEEP if available, but do not be afraid to increase pressures to 30 cmH$_2$O after checking airway positioning if there is no heart rate response. Any very obvious chest wall movement in babies

Table 10.1 Acceptable oxygen saturations after birth.

Time from birth (min)	Acceptable (25th centile) preductal saturation (%)
2	60
3	70
4	80
5	85
10	90

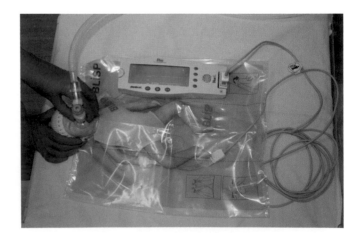

Figure 10.4 Premature baby manikin in plastic bag with saturation probe attached.

of <28 weeks gestation may indicate excessive, and potentially damaging, tidal volumes.

Premature babies are more susceptible to the toxic effects of hyperoxia. Using a pulse oximeter to monitor both heart rate and oxygen makes stabilisation much easier. Ranges of preductal oxygen saturation found in the first few minutes of life in well preterm infants are increasingly being reported; however, only small numbers are from well babies born before 32 weeks gestation. Additional oxygen should not be given if the oxygen saturation from the right arm or wrist exceeds the values in Table 10.1.

Saturation monitoring

Pulse oximetry gives a quick and relatively accurate display of both heart rate and oxygen saturation, which can be easily seen by all involved in the resuscitation. This is particularly useful when stabilising significantly preterm babies (Figure 10.4) or when considering additional oxygen in any baby. Once the heart rate is displayed it is likely that this will be more accurate than other commonly used methods of assessing heart rate.

Further reading

Kattwinkel J, Perlman JM, Aziz K, *et al*. Part 15: Neonatal Resuscitation: 2010. American Heart Association Guidelines for Cardiopulmonary Resuscitation and Emergency Cardiovascular Care. *Circulation* 2010;**122**;S909–19

Richmond S (ed.). *Newborn Life Support* (3rd edn). London, Resuscitation Council (UK), 2010.

Richmond S, Wyllie J. European Resuscitation Council Guidelines for Resuscitation 2010. Section 7. Resuscitation of babies at birth. *Resuscitation* **2010**:81;1219–76.

Richmond S, Wyllie J. Newborn life support. In Nolan JP (ed.). *2010 Resuscitation Guidelines* pp. 118–27. London, 2010, Resuscitation Council (UK). Available at http://www.resus.org.uk/pages/nls.pdf.

Saugstad OD. New guidelines for newborn resuscitation – a critical evaluation. *Acta Paediatr* 2011;**100**:1058–62.

Wyllie J, Perlman JM, Kattwinkel J, *et al*. Part 11: neonatal resuscitation: 2010 International Consensus on Cardiopulmonary Resuscitation and Emergency Cardiovascular Care Science With Treatment Recommendations. *Resuscitation* 2010:**81S**;e260–87.

CHAPTER 11

Out-of-Hospital Resuscitation

Joanne K. Smith[1], Mark Whitbread[1] and Fionna P. Moore[1,2]

[1]London Ambulance Service NHS Trust, London, UK
[2]Imperial College Healthcare Trust, London, UK

OVERVIEW

- Early recognition of cardiac arrest, calling an ambulance and immediate bystander CPR improve survival from out-of-hospital cardiac arrest

- Automated external defibrillator (AED) use by responders before ambulance arrival improves survival from ventricular fibrillation/pulseless ventricular tachycardia cardiac arrest

- Ambulance service dispatchers provide telephone instructions to untrained bystanders on how to do chest compressions

- Paramedics are trained and equipped to deliver advanced life support treatments at the scene

- Effective CPR during transport is difficult – when feasible, the aim is to achieve a return of spontaneous circulation at the scene and stabilise the patient before hospital transfer

- Transfer to a hospital capable of providing comprehensive post-resuscitation care that includes primary angioplasty and therapeutic hypothermia is associated with improved survival

- Recognition of Life Extinct (ROLE) guidance helps prevent futile resuscitation attempts

Introduction

Out-of-hospital sudden death is a leading cause of death in the industrialised world. In Europe alone, 700,000 sudden cardiac arrests occur each year. There is marked variation in the incidence of and outcomes from out-of-hospital cardiac arrest between and within countries. This was highlighted in a recent systematic review that found 10-fold variation in incidence and outcomes for out-of-hospital cardiac arrest. In the UK, analysis of early data from the National Ambulance Quality Indicators shows variation in return of spontaneous circulation (ROSC) rates (13.3–26.7%) and survival to hospital discharge (2.2–12%). The sources of such variation may be related to the data (e.g. case and data definitions), patient (e.g. co-morbidities, age), environmental (e.g. location of arrest, whether it was witnessed, whether bystander CPR is commenced), EMS process variables (EMS response time, quality of CPR) and hospital variables (e.g. use of therapeutic

ABC of Resuscitation, Sixth Edition. Edited by Jasmeet Soar, Gavin D. Perkins and Jerry Nolan.
© 2013 John Wiley & Sons, Ltd. Published 2013 by John Wiley & Sons, Ltd.

hypothermia and percutaneous coronary intervention facilities). A systems approach covering the whole patient journey may help standardise and improve outcomes.

Emergency Medical System (EMS) response

The case for providing prompt and effective resuscitation at the scene of an emergency is overwhelming and a variety of emergency care roles exist in the pre-hospital arena. The majority of acutely unwell patients seeking help will most commonly receive a response in the form of a double manned ambulance staffed by paramedics and/or emergency medical technicians (EMTs). In many areas, single responders in a car, motorcycle or pushbike are used increasingly to undertake initial assessment and treatment. Many paramedics have developed their clinical practice into specialist and advanced roles in both primary and critical care. These roles include paramedic practitioner, emergency care practitioner, critical care paramedic and consultant paramedic, operating not only in ambulance services but also with out-of-hours GP providers, in minor injury units and walk-in centres. In order to practice, all paramedics must now register with the Health Professions Council (HPC) and their education is moving towards the higher education model.

EMS dispatch

Emergency calls are categorised depending on the condition of the patient. The highest priority, 'category A', is reserved for patients with an immediately life-threatening condition such as cardiac arrest, chest pain, severe difficulty in breathing, time-critical stroke or severe haemorrhage. It is standard practice for a rapid response unit (in the form of a car, motorbike or even pushbike) to be sent as an initial resource prior to the arrival of an ambulance to undertake initial assessment and treatment. Figure 11.1 illustrates typical frontline responses, one or more of which may be dispatched to a 999 call.

Other pre-hospital providers include air ambulance teams and BASICS doctors. The nature of calls that air ambulances are dispatched to depends considerably on the geographical area. For example, in London there is one air ambulance which attends major trauma. In more remote regions of the country, helicopters

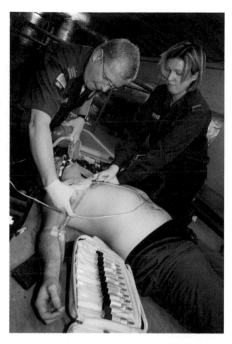

Figure 11.1 Paramedic crew performing advanced life support.

may be dispatched to 'medically unwell' patients, for instance those suffering a heart attack or stroke. BASICS doctors are specialists that have received specific training on how to work outside the hospital environment. They provide specialist support to augment the ambulance service response.

Initial assessment

On arrival at the scene, paramedics will perform an assessment of the patient to identify their immediate healthcare needs. This may involve making critical decisions regarding treatment and may include performing life-saving interventions before triaging the patient to an appropriate centre. The remit of the standard paramedic role may include managing any medical or trauma-related incident from abdominal pain to a multi-patient road traffic collision. Box 11.1 lists the conditions where paramedics can play a vital part.

Box 11.1 **List of conditions where paramedics can play a vital part**

- Cardiac/respiratory arrest
- Acute coronary syndromes (ACS)
- Stroke
- Asthma, chronic obstructive pulmonary disease
- Heart failure
- Obstetric emergencies
- Trauma
- Diabetic emergencies
- Airway obstruction
- Drug overdose
- Life threatening cardiac arrhythmias
- Anaphylaxis

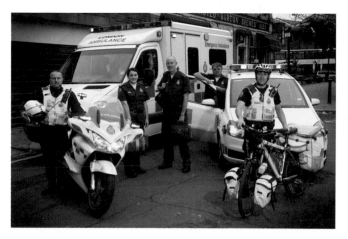

Figure 11.2 The range of frontline responses, one or more of which may be dispatched to an emergency call.

Pre-hospital interventions

Paramedics are trained to perform advanced life support (ALS) and a range of life-saving interventions (see Box 11.2). Figure 11.2 depicts a paramedic crew performing ALS in the pre-hospital environment. Paramedics may deliver a wide range of drugs, the majority of which are set out in Box 11.3. Specialist paramedics may also prescribe and administer a range of drugs under 'patient group directions' which previously may only have been prescribed by a GP or in hospital.

Box 11.2 **Paramedic skill set**

- Basic airway management and ventilation
- Supraglottic airway insertion
- Endotracheal intubation
- Needle cricothyroidotomy
- Needle thoracocentesis
- Intravenous and intra-osseous cannulation

Box 11.3 **Drugs sanctioned for use by paramedics**

- Adrenaline
- Atropine
- Aspirin
- Benzylpenicillin
- Chlorphenamine
- Diazepam
- Glucagon
- Glyceryl trinitrate (GTN)
- Hydrocortisone
- Ipratropium bromide
- Morphine
- Naloxone
- Nitrous oxide
- Sodium chloride
- Syntometrine
- Thrombolytic agents
- Paracetamol
- Dexamethasone
- Ibuprofen

Performance

Until recently, UK ambulance services were solely measured on their performance by their ability to reach patients rapidly, in particular, 75% of category A calls within 8 minutes. The Department of Health (DH) has now introduced a number of 'clinical indicators' and ambulance services are now, in addition to response time targets, measured on clinical indicators including cardiac arrest survival rate and percentage of ST segment elevation myocardial infarction (STEMI) and stroke patients conveyed to specialist centres. Ambulance services are, in addition, measured on their delivery of 'care bundles' for certain conditions such as ACS and stroke.

National guidelines

The guidelines for patient care to which ambulance clinicians are expected to adhere are set out by the Joint Royal Colleges Ambulance Liaison Committee (JRCALC). JRCALC has representatives nominated by their respective specialities/colleges. Its role is to provide robust clinical speciality advice to ambulance services. Although all ambulance services have endorsed these guidelines, there are variations on some that have been agreed by the ambulance service clinical lead.

Chain of survival

The key therapeutic interventions of the chain of survival (Figure 11.3) are characterised as early access, early CPR, early defibrillation, early ALS and timely post-resuscitation care. Additional factors, including whether the collapse was witnessed, the presenting cardiac rhythm and co-morbidity are associated with the likelihood of successful resuscitation.

Early access

This initial link of the chain relates to the early recognition of cardiac arrest and an early call for help. Campaigns over recent years highlighting the signs and symptoms of heart attack (e.g. 'Doubt Kills' campaign; Figure 11.4) aim to improve public awareness.

The UK has a dedicated emergency number, 999, which anyone in need of emergency assistance may access. 112, the number used across Europe, may also be used in the UK. Call takers receiving the 999 calls are not medically trained and follow a standard set of instructions (Figures 11.5 and 11.6). All services use MPDS (Medical

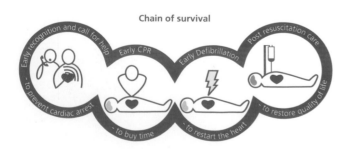

Figure 11.3 Chain of survival.

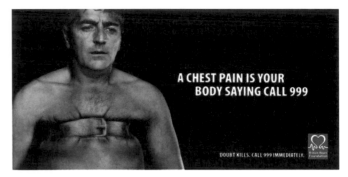

Figure 11.4 The BHF's 'Doubt Kills' campaign. Reproduced with the permission of the British Heart Foundation.

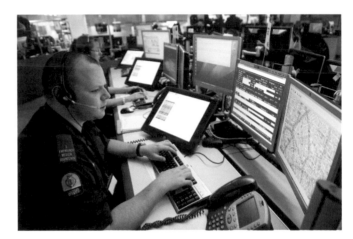

Figure 11.5 Emergency medical dispatcher in control room.

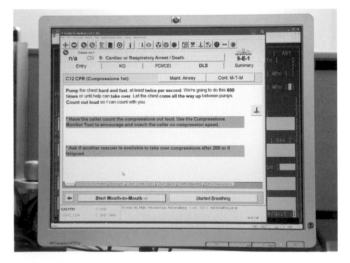

Figure 11.6 Dispatch life support instructions delivered in control room by 999 call takers.

Priority Dispatch System) or NHS Pathways, which rapidly categorise calls received into order of priority depending on the patient's symptoms; resources can then be allocated and dispatched. These resources may include Community First Responders (CFRs), Public Access Defibrillation (PAD) sites, as well as conventional ambulance responses.

Early CPR

Patients who receive early CPR have an increased survival – twice that of those who do not. Despite this, only one-third of out-of-hospital cardiac arrest victims receive bystander CPR. In the event of a patient identified as 'not breathing' during the emergency call to the ambulance, call takers provide telephone-assisted CPR instructions. Dispatch life support for patients in suspected cardiac arrest omits ventilations and the rescuer is guided towards providing 'chest compression only CPR'.

All frontline emergency staff are trained in CPR and paramedics in ALS. All UK ambulance services use trained CFRs, volunteers from the local community, equipped with basic resuscitation equipment including automated external defibrillators (AEDs) and oxygen. These volunteers are able to deliver CPR and defibrillation prior to the arrival of the emergency services.

Most ambulance services offer training to the public in emergency life support skills. 'Heartstart' training, a scheme led by the British Heart Foundation, encourages education in CPR skills and provides organisations such as schools with the necessary equipment to deliver CPR training; 2.9 million people have now been trained in emergency life-saving skills through this scheme.

Early defibrillation

The importance of early defibrillation cannot be emphasised enough for those patients who present in a shockable rhythm. All frontline ambulances across the UK carry defibrillators, either in the form of AEDs, larger defibrillator monitors or both.

Early defibrillation is a key element in the chain of survival and it has now become a challenge to further reduce the time from cardiac arrest to defibrillation by EMS personnel. One method of reducing this 'time to first defibrillatory shock' is to encourage laypeople to administer defibrillation using an AED. The British Heart Foundation has subsidised AEDs in public places since the early 1990s, and most ambulance services are now responsible for some form of public access defibrillation (PAD) programme. AEDs are commonly sited in major transport hubs including airports, train and underground stations, shopping centres, tourist attractions, schools and sports centres. The Resuscitation Council (UK) recommends that any member of the public, if willing, is permitted to use an AED in the event of a suspected cardiac arrest, even if the rescuer is untrained. AEDs are extremely easy to use and will only deliver a shock to a patient who is in a 'shockable rhythm'. Survival from PAD sites is frequently high, and rates as high as 74% have been reported.

Early advanced life support

Paramedics can deliver ALS through airway management and intravenous access for drugs and fluid administration. Increasingly, the emphasis during training and practice is now placed on good basic airway management and the use of supraglottic airways for obtunded patients rather than endotracheal intubation.

Much emphasis is placed on the importance of recording end tidal carbon dioxide ($ETCO_2$) immediately following placement of either a supraglottic airway or an endotracheal tube to confirm correct positioning. $ETCO_2$ measurement may also provide valuable feedback about the effectiveness of the CPR being performed.

Post-resuscitation care

Stabilisation and monitoring

Every effort should be made to stabilise patients on scene as much as practically possible before transportation whilst avoiding unnecessary delays. Evidence suggests that removal prior to stabilisation is likely to result in ineffective compressions and failed resuscitation. Stabilisation may include the acquisition and interpretation of a 12-lead ECG, administration of fluid and atropine as well as advanced airway management (Figure 11.7).

Therapeutic interventions

Ideally, patients should be conveyed to a centre capable of performing primary angioplasty, therapeutic hypothermia and with full intensive care capacity. The concept of 'cardiac arrest centres' is only in its embryonic stages in the UK but may provide a basis for the future of intra- and post-cardiac arrest care. Already, in some ambulance services, patients who display ST elevation on their post-arrest 12-lead ECG are conveyed direct to Heart Attack Centres regardless of their level of consciousness.

Mild therapeutic hypothermia is neuroprotective and has been demonstrated to improve outcome after a period of global cerebral hypoxia/ischaemia. Cooling should start as soon as possible after ROSC.

Termination of resuscitation attempts

The 'Recognition of Life Extinct' (ROLE) procedure describes the circumstances where initiation of resuscitation is inappropriate or where resuscitation performed by paramedics and EMTs may be terminated (Figure 11.8). A Medical Certificate for the Cause of Death (MCCD) may subsequently be issued by a medical practitioner or HM Coroner.

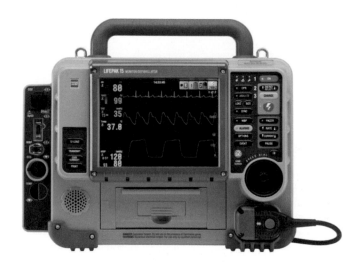

Figure 11.7 Example of monitor defibrillator typically used to obtain a 12-lead ECG and measure end tidal carbon dioxide.

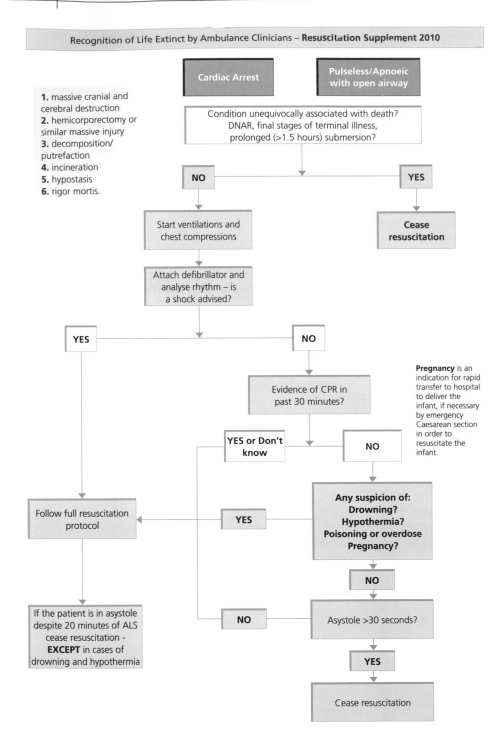

Recognition of Life Extinct by Ambulance Clinicians – **Resuscitation Supplement 2010**

Cardiac Arrest

Pulseless/Apnoeic with open airway

1. massive cranial and cerebral destruction
2. hemicorporectomy or similar massive injury
3. decomposition/putrefaction
4. incineration
5. hypostasis
6. rigor mortis.

Condition unequivocally associated with death? DNAR, final stages of terminal illness, prolonged (>1.5 hours) submersion?

NO

YES

Start ventilations and chest compressions

Cease resuscitation

Attach defibrillator and analyse rhythm – is a shock advised?

YES

NO

Evidence of CPR in past 30 minutes?

Pregnancy is an indication for rapid transfer to hospital to deliver the infant, if necessary by emergency Caesarean section in order to resuscitate the infant.

YES or Don't know

NO

Follow full resuscitation protocol

Any suspicion of: Drowning? Hypothermia? Poisoning or overdose Pregnancy?

YES

NO

If the patient is in asystole despite 20 minutes of ALS cease resuscitation - **EXCEPT** in cases of drowning and hypothermia

NO

Asystole >30 seconds?

YES

Cease resuscitation

Figure 11.8 Recognition of Life Extinct by Ambulance Clinicians Algorithm. Reproduced from the *UK Ambulance Services Clinical Practice Guidelines* (Fisher *et al.* 2012) (www.warwick.ac.uk/go/jrcalcguidelines).

Further reading

Fisher JD, Brown SN, Cooke MW (Eds). *UK Ambulance Services Clinical Practice Guidelines (2012)*. Class Publishing Ltd, 2012.

Jewkes F, Nolan JP. Resuscitation Council (UK) Pre-hospital cardiac arrest. 2010. http://www.resus.org.uk/pages/prehosca.pdf

Neumar RW, Barnhart JM, Berg RA *et al*. Implementation strategies for improving survival after out-of-hospital cardiac arrest in the United States: Consensus recommendations from the 2009 American Heart Association Cardiac Arrest Survival Summit, *Circulation* 2011;**123**:2898–910.

Nichol G, Aufderheide TP, Eigel B, *et al*. Regional systems of care for out-of-hospital cardiac arrest: A policy statement from the American Heart Association. *Circulation* 2010;**121**(5):709–29.

Olasveengen TM, Wik L, Steen PA. Quality of cardiopulmonary resuscitation before and during transport in out-of-hospital cardiac arrest. *Resuscitation* 2008;**76**(2):185–90.

CHAPTER 12

In-Hospital CPR

Robin P. Davies[1] and Gavin D. Perkins[1,2]

[1]Heart Of England NHS Foundation Trust, Birmingham, UK
[2]Warwick Medical School, University of Warwick, Coventry, UK

OVERVIEW

- Hospitals must be able to provide a resilient response to in-hospital cardiac arrest
- All clinical staff should be able to recognise cardiac arrest, know how to activate the emergency resuscitation team and be able to initiate emergency treatment whilst awaiting arrival of the resuscitation team
- Initial treatment should focus on delivery of high-quality, uninterrupted chest compressions
- Local responders should provide a focused handover when the resuscitation team arrives
- Mock cardiac arrest drills usefully test the emergency response

Introduction

Patients and their relatives expect a prompt, effective response to in-hospital cardiac arrest. All clinical staff must be able to recognise the physiological and clinical signs of deterioration and respond promptly in the event of cardiac arrest occurring. Chapter 3 describes how to recognise a patient at risk of cardiac arrest and how to intervene in an attempt to prevent a cardiac arrest from occurring. If cardiac arrest has occurred, in most hospital settings (e.g. ward, clinics, operating theatres) clinical staff are expected to call for help and initiate resuscitation. Definitive care is then provided by a resuscitation team with staff trained and skilled in advanced life support (ALS) techniques.

Recognising cardiac arrest

Assess the patient for a response: ask the patient, 'Are you all right?' If there is no response, gently shake their shoulders; if the patient does not respond, shout for help/activate the emergency call buzzer. Open the airway using the head tilt, chin lift manoeuvre. Keeping the airway open, look, listen and feel for normal breathing and other signs of life. If trained to do so, palpate the carotid pulse

ABC of Resuscitation, Sixth Edition. Edited by Jasmeet Soar, Gavin D. Perkins and Jerry Nolan.
© 2013 John Wiley & Sons, Ltd. Published 2013 by John Wiley & Sons, Ltd.

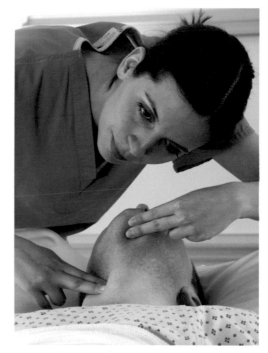

Figure 12.1 Confirming cardiac arrest by feeling for a carotid pulse and simultaneously checking for a pulse. Photograph reproduced with kind permission by Michael Scott and the Resuscitation Council (UK).

simultaneously (Figure 12.1). Take no more than 10 s to assess breathing/pulse. If the patient has no signs of life (confirmed by absence of normal breathing, coughing, purposeful movement), or there is doubt, start CPR and call the resuscitation team. Figure 12.2 summarises the sequence of steps for the initial assessment of the collapsed patient.

Agonal breathing

Do not confuse agonal breathing, a brainstem response to hypoxia, with normal breathing. It is common in the early stages of cardiac arrest and should not be confused with signs of life. Agonal breathing may also start during CPR as cerebral perfusion improves, but it does not indicate return of spontaneous circulation (ROSC). Agonal breathing has a characteristic pattern (Box 12.1) and should be recognised as a sign of cardiac arrest.

In-hospital Resuscitation Algorithm

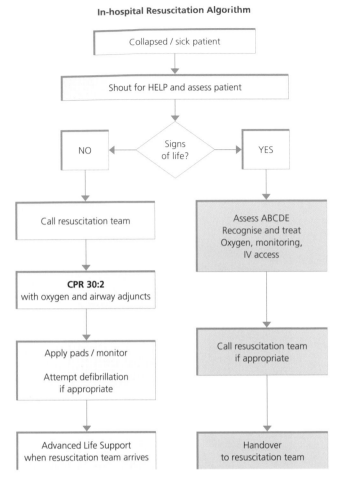

Figure 12.2 Initial sequence of steps for the assessment and treatment of the collapsed patient. Reproduced with the kind permission of the Resuscitation Council (UK).

Box 12.1 Common descriptions of agonal breathing (data from Clark et al. 1992)

- Barely breathing
- Heavy breathing
- Laboured breathing
- Problems breathing
- Noisy breathing
- Gasping breathing

Start resuscitation

Start resuscitation by delivering 30 high-quality chest compressions (Figure 12.3). Chest compressions should be to a depth of 5–6 cm, at a rate of 100–120 min^{-1}. If performing CPR on a mattress, push deeper to compensate for compression of the underlying mattress. Allow full chest recoil between each chest compression. After 30 chest compressions, give 2 ventilations using a bag-mask or barrier device (Figure 12.4a and b). Add supplemental oxygen as soon as available. Continue sequences of 30 compressions to 2 ventilations. If there are delays in delivering ventilations, continue chest compressions alone until this can be rectified.

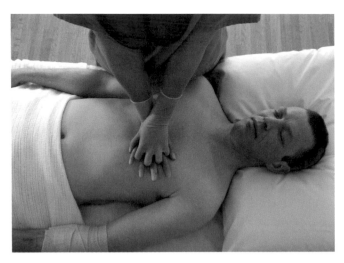

Figure 12.3 To deliver high-quality chest compressions, place the hands in the centre of the chest (between the nipples), compress the chest 5–6 cm in depth, at a rate of 100–120 min^{-1}. Allow the chest to fully recoil between compressions. Photograph reproduced with kind permission by Michael Scott and the Resuscitation Council (UK).

Activate the emergency resuscitation team

Once CPR is in progress, call for the resuscitation team. In the UK a standardised emergency telephone number is used – 2222. This number is often also used to activate other emergency teams, for example trauma, paediatric, obstetric, neonatal, fire, security. Ensure that clear instructions are provided to the person who is sent to call the resuscitation team. Avoid the use of terms that may cause confusion such as 'the patient has crashed', 'put out the call', or 'code blue'. Switchboard operators are not clinically trained and can respond only to the information provided by the caller. The person making the 2222 call must therefore state clearly the location of the emergency and the response required (Figure 12.5). Errors in communication are common and can lead to delays in activating the emergency team (Box 12.2).

Box 12.2 Common communication errors when placing an emergency 2222 call

- Providing unnecessary detail, e.g. patient name, reason for admission, sequence of events prior to arrest
- Failing to speak clearly – talking too quickly, hesitancy, pronounced accents
- Caller uncertain of nature of emergency/response required
- Caller uncertain of location of emergency
- Imprecise terminology, e.g. call the 'crash team'; 'code blue'

Continue high-quality CPR

Continue high-quality CPR while the resuscitation team is en route. Consider the use of simple airway adjuncts such as an oral or nasal pharyngeal airway to aid airway management and therefore ventilation. Consider insertion of a supraglottic airway (SAD) (e.g. laryngeal mask airway or i-gel), as it provides more effective

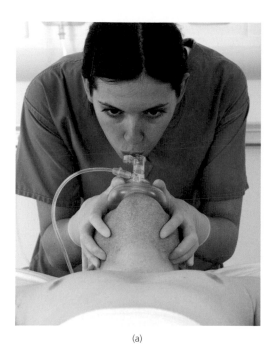
(a)

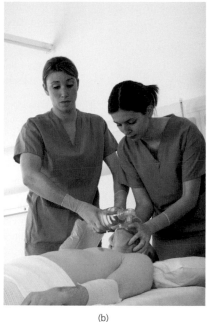
(b)

Figure 12.4 After 30 compressions, provide 2 ventilations using (a) a barrier device or (b) bag-mask device. Photograph reproduced with kind permission by Michael Scott and the Resuscitation Council (UK).

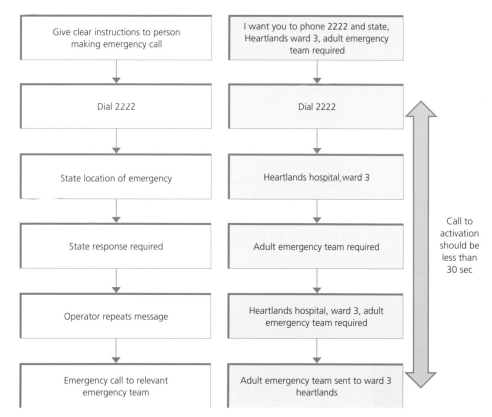

Figure 12.5 Provide clear and concise information to the telephone operator.

ventilation than a bag-mask device alone. Tracheal intubation is a complex procedure and should only be undertaken by fully trained staff with regular and ongoing exposure to intubation. Minimise interruptions to chest compressions during the placement of the device. Once a definitive airway (SAD or tracheal tube) is in place, switch to continuous chest compressions while providing

ventilation without pausing chest compressions at a rate of about 10 breaths min^{-1}. If a SAD is in place, check that ventilation is adequate; if not, return to delivering CPR at a ratio of 30:2

Attempt to obtain intravenous access if not already available. Consider intra-osseous access if intravenous access cannot be obtained quickly. Obtain the patient's medical notes and drug treatment record. Do not allow any of these interventions to interrupt CPR.

Defibrillation

Prompt delivery of a shock within 2–3 min of the onset of ventricular fibrillation/ventricular tachycardia (VF/VT) is associated with improved outcomes. Hospitals should ensure that every clinical area has access to a defibrillator within these timeframes. There are two different types of external defibrillators: (a) manual defibrillators require the defibrillator operator to interpret the ECG trace and determine if the rhythm is shockable; (b) semi-automatic or automated external defibrillators (AEDs) automate the process of cardiac rhythm analysis (Figure 12.6). Some defibrillators can operate in either manual or semi-automatic mode.

Semi-automatic/AEDs use complex pattern recognition algorithms to recognise shockable rhythms with a minimum sensitivity (correct identification of a shockable rhythm) of >90% and specificity (correct identification that the rhythm is non-shockable) of >95%. The time taken to identify the underlying rhythm, charge the capacitor and deliver a shock can range from a few seconds to over a minute. This can cause prolonged periods of no flow while chest compressions are paused. Whilst undoubtedly lifesaving outside hospitals, recent studies have suggested that the in-hospital use of AEDs may be linked to worse outcomes, particularly if the initial rhythm is non-shockable.

Pending definitive trials, a sensible approach is for the ward team to focus initially on high-quality, uninterrupted CPR. If staff are trained in manual defibrillation and a person is available, use this in preference to an AED. If an AED is the only option, deploy it only after high-quality CPR has been commenced. When the resuscitation team arrives, switch the AED to manual mode or change over to a manual defibrillator.

Handover to the resuscitation team

When the resuscitation team arrives, continue CPR and provide a brief synopsis of events. Use of a structure communication tool (e.g. SBAR – Situation–Background–Assessment–Recommendation) is helpful (Box 12.3). After this briefing, decide who will continue as arrest team leader. Ward staff should continue to provide support to

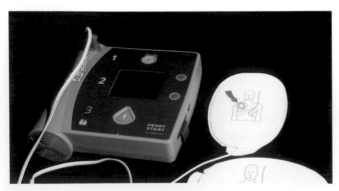

Figure 12.6 Automated external defibrillator.

the resuscitation team. They must also check that there is sufficient cover to ensure the health and safety of other patients.

> **Box 12.3 Example of the use of SBAR tool for handover to the resuscitation team**
>
> - Situation: Mr Smith sustained a witnessed cardiac arrest approximately 3 minutes ago
> - Background: He is 55 years old and was admitted 24 hours ago with shortness of breath thought to be secondary to community acquired pneumonia. He was previously fit and healthy. He is receiving intravenous antibiotics and DVT prophylaxis with low molecular weight heparin
> - Assessment: We started CPR immediately. We have obtained intravenous access and are giving him 500 ml of normal saline
> - Recommendation: Are you ready for me to handover managing his arrest to you at the end of this cycle?

Resuscitation team

Most hospitals provide a designated resuscitation team. This team may also serve other roles such as that of a medical emergency team. The team should comprise 4–6 people with the necessary training and clinical skills to manage a cardiac arrest (Box 12.4). All clinical members of the resuscitation team should be qualified in advanced resuscitation skills (e.g. the ALS or Immediate Life Support (ILS) certificate). Some specialist high-dependency areas (e.g. emergency department, critical care unit, coronary care) may have sufficient staff with advanced skills to manage arrests in-house without calling a separate resuscitation team. Resuscitation teams should meet at the start of each shift and pre-assign roles prior to being called to an emergency. Immediate (hot debrief) or post-event debriefing may improve future team performance and reduce stress amongst the team.

> **Box 12.4 Cardiac arrest team roles**
>
> - Team leader
> - Airway
> - CPR
> - Vascular access
> - Drug preparation and administration
> - Defibrillation
> - Runner

Planning for the emergency response

Hospitals should have clear policies and procedures for managing a patient in cardiac arrest. This will include details of the necessary training for staff, provision of emergency equipment and how to get help. In most situations this will involve activating an internal resuscitation team. In remote locations or in areas where a resuscitation team is not available it will be necessary to call an ambulance.

Table 12.1 Suggested emergency equipment.

Advanced airway	Breathing	Circulation	Drugs	Miscellaneous
Suction	Pocket mask	Defibrillator	Adrenaline	Sharps box
Oxygen + mask	Bag-mask device	Intravenous cannulae	Amiodarone	Gloves
Oropharyngeal airways		(various sizes)	Glucose	Audit form
Nasopharyngeal airways		IO needle/device	Fluids	Drip stand
Supraglottic airways		Giving sets	Atropine	Various size syringes
Equipment for intubation			Calcium chloride	Arterial blood gas
			Magnesium	syringes

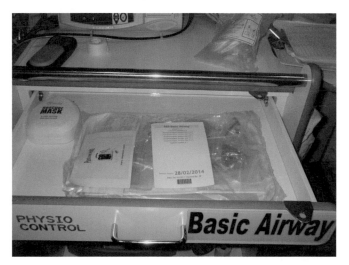

Figure 12.7 Basic airway tray in a drawer of a standardised resuscitation trolley.

Clinical staff training

Clinical staff should be able to recognise cardiac arrest, activate the emergency team and initiate resuscitation. In higher risk areas (e.g. operating suites, critical care units) more advanced skills (e.g. defibrillation, vascular access, airway management) may be required. Even though skill decay is seen within a few weeks of training, current guidelines only require staff to be updated in CPR skills at least once a year. Regular skill updates within the workplace (rolling refreshers) enable staff to maintain their competence between annual updates.

Equipment

Standardised resuscitation equipment should be immediately available to all clinical areas (Table 12.1). The readiness of equipment for use should be checked daily. The use of sealed trolleys prevents the inappropriate use of emergency equipment for routine procedures (Figure 12.7) and reduces the burden of daily inspections and equipment errors.

Emergency drills

Emergency activation systems (e.g. pager systems) should be tested at least once a day. Response rates to the daily test call should be regularly audited. Mock emergencies/mock arrests provide a safe way to test the resilience of the emergency response. Such drills allow staff to familiarise themselves with the emergency response system and their roles and enables telephone, pager, team response times and completeness to be tested.

Further reading

Akhtar N, Field R, Greenwood E, *et al.* Quality of in-hospital cardiac arrest calls: a prospective observational study. *BMJ Qual Saf* 2012;**21**(3):184–90.

Clark JJ, Larsen MP, Culley LL, Graves JR, Eisenberg MS. Incidence of agonal respirations in sudden cardiac arrest. *Ann Emerg Med* 1992;**21**(12):1464–7.

Deakin C, Nolan JP, Perkins GD, Lockey AS. Resuscitation Council (UK) Adult Advanced Life Support Guidelines, 2010. http://www.resus.org.uk/pages/als.pdf

Deakin CD, Morrison LJ, Morley PT, *et al.* Advanced Life Support Chapter Collaborators. Part 8: Advanced life support: 2010 International Consensus on Cardiopulmonary Resuscitation and Emergency Cardiovascular Care Science with Treatment Recommendations. *Resuscitation* 2010;**81**(Suppl 1):e93–e174.

Niles D, Sutton RM, Donoghue A, *et al.* 'Rolling refreshers': a novel approach to maintain CPR psychomotor skill competence. *Resuscitation* 2009;**80**:909–12.

Perkins GD, Kocierz L, Smith SC, McCulloch RA, Davies RP. Compression feedback devices overestimate chest compression depth when performed on a bed. *Resuscitation* 2009;**80**:79–82.

Soar J, Davies RP. In hospital CPR. http://www.resus.org.uk/pages/inhresus.pdf

CHAPTER 13

Peri-arrest Arrhythmias

Jerry Nolan[1] and David Pitcher[2]

[1]Royal United Hospital, Bath, UK
[2]University Hospital Birmingham, UK

OVERVIEW

- Some arrhythmias may occur prior to cardiac arrest – recognition and appropriate treatment of an arrhythmia with adverse features may prevent progression to cardiac arrest
- Arrhythmias occurring after resuscitation from cardiac arrest and ROSC may need treatment to stabilise the patient and prevent recurrence of cardiac arrest
- The urgency for treatment and the best choice of treatment is determined by the condition of the patient (presence or absence of adverse features) and by the nature and cause of the arrhythmia
- Assessment of a patient with an arrhythmia follows the ABCDE approach.
- Whenever possible the arrhythmia should be documented on a 12-lead ECG

Introduction

Arrhythmias are common in the peri-arrest period: they may lead to cardiac arrest or they may occur soon after return of spontaneous circulation (ROSC), a time when the myocardium is frequently 'electrically unstable'. Arrhythmias that may lead to cardiac arrest or to avoidable deterioration in the patient's condition require urgent treatment; others may require no immediate treatment. When an arrhythmia is present or suspected, the patient is first assessed using the ABCDE approach, which will include applying an ECG monitor and, whenever possible, recording a 12-lead ECG. The patient is assessed for presence or absence of adverse features and an attempt is made to diagnose the arrhythmia.

All defibrillator energy levels given in this chapter refer to biphasic waveforms.

Adverse features

The presence or absence of adverse symptoms or signs will dictate the urgency and choice of treatment for most arrhythmias (Box 13.1).

ABC of Resuscitation, Sixth Edition. Edited by Jasmeet Soar, Gavin D. Perkins and Jerry Nolan.
© 2013 John Wiley & Sons, Ltd. Published 2013 by John Wiley & Sons, Ltd.

Box 13.1 **Adverse features indicating a potentially 'unstable' patient**

- Shock – Hypotension (systolic blood pressure <90 mmHg), pallor, sweating, cold, extremities, confusion or impaired consciousness
- Syncope
- Heart failure
- Myocardial ischaemia – chest pain and/or evidence of myocardial ischaemia on 12-lead ECG
- Extremes of heart rate: tachycardia >150 min^{-1}; bradycardia <40 min^{-1}

In general, the presence of adverse features implies the need for more rapid treatment: in some cases, a simple clinical intervention, such as a vagal manoeuvre, may be effective but more commonly there is some form of electrical intervention (cardioversion for tachyarrhythmia or pacing for bradyarrhythmia). In the absence of adverse features, assuming treatment is indicated, the use of drugs is usually appropriate.

If a patient develops an arrhythmia as a complication of some other condition (e.g. infection, acute myocardial infarction, heart failure), that condition is assessed and treated as appropriate.

Tachyarrhythmia

The adult tachycardia algorithm is shown in Figure 13.1.

Tachycardia with adverse features

The presence of adverse features implies that the patient's condition is unstable and the preferred treatment is likely to be synchronised cardioversion. Although a heart rate of >150 min^{-1} is considered an adverse sign, patients with impaired cardiac function, structural heart disease or other serious medical conditions may be symptomatic with heart rates between 100 and 150 min^{-1}.

Synchronised cardioversion

Before cardioversion is attempted, the patient will need to be anaesthetised or sedated by a healthcare professional with the appropriate competencies.

Set the defibrillator to deliver a synchronised shock; this delivers the shock to coincide with the R wave. An unsynchronised shock could coincide with a T wave and cause ventricular fibrillation (VF).

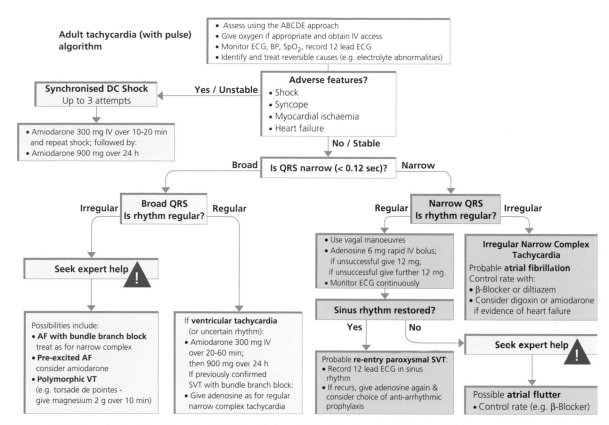

Figure 13.1 The adult tachycardia algorithm. Reproduced with the kind permission of the Resuscitation Council (UK).

For a broad-complex tachycardia or atrial fibrillation, start with 120–150 J and increase in increments if this fails. Atrial flutter and regular narrow-complex tachycardia will often be terminated by lower-energy shocks; therefore, start with 70–120 J.

If cardioversion fails to terminate the arrhythmia, and adverse features persist, give amiodarone 300 mg i.v. over 10–20 min and attempt further synchronised cardioversion. The loading dose of amiodarone can be followed by an infusion of 900 mg over 24 h given preferably via a central vein.

Tachycardia without adverse features

If there are no adverse features, consider treatment with a drug. Some anti-arrhythmic drugs may cause myocardial depression or another tachyarrhythmia, or provoke severe bradycardia.

Broad-complex tachycardia

Broad-complex tachycardia (QRS ≥ 0.12 s) may be ventricular in origin or may be a supraventricular rhythm with aberrant conduction (i.e. bundle branch block). In the patient with adverse features, the distinction is irrelevant – the treatment is to attempt synchronised cardioversion. In the absence of adverse features, next determine whether the rhythm is regular or irregular.

Regular broad-complex tachycardia

A regular broad-complex tachycardia may be ventricular tachycardia (VT) (Figure 13.2) or supraventricular tachycardia (SVT) with bundle branch block. In a stable patient, adenosine, when given during a continuous, multi-lead ECG recording, may help to determine the rhythm by causing AV block and demonstrating the underlying atrial rhythm if the rhythm is of supraventricular origin. If the rhythm is VT, adenosine will have no effect on heart rhythm or rate. If VT, give amiodarone 300 mg i.v. over 20–60 min, followed by 900 mg over 24 h. If a regular broad-complex tachycardia is known to be SVT with bundle branch block, and the patient is stable, treat as for narrow-complex tachycardia.

Irregular broad-complex tachycardia

This is most likely to be atrial fibrillation (AF) with bundle branch block but less common causes are AF with ventricular pre-excitation (in patients with Wolff–Parkinson–White (WPW) syndrome), or

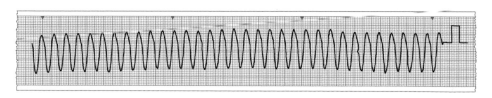

Figure 13.2 Monomorphic ventricular tachycardia. Copyright © 2012 Dr Oliver Meyer, Reproduced with permission.

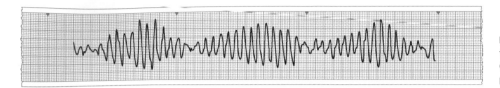

Figure 13.3 Polymorphic ventricular tachycardia – *torsade de pointes*. Copyright © 2012 Dr Oliver Meyer, Reproduced with permission.

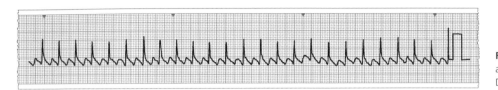

Figure 13.4 Atrial flutter with 2:1 atrioventricular block. Copyright © 2012 Dr Oliver Meyer, Reproduced with permission.

polymorphic VT (e.g. *torsade de pointes*) (Figure 13.3). Polymorphic VT is likely to be associated with adverse features.

If the rhythm is *torsade de pointes*, stop all drugs known to prolong the QT interval, correct electrolyte abnormalities (especially hypokalaemia) and give magnesium sulphate 2 g i.v. over 10 min. Once the arrhythmia has been corrected, seek expert help because overdrive pacing may be indicated to prevent relapse. If adverse features develop, which is common, give a shock. If the patient becomes pulseless, attempt defibrillation immediately and follow the cardiac arrest algorithm.

Narrow-complex tachycardia

Regular narrow-complex tachycardias include sinus tachycardia, atrioventricular nodal re-entry tachycardia (AVNRT; the commonest type of regular narrow-complex tachyarrhythmia), atrioventricular re-entry tachycardia (AVRT; due to WPW syndrome) and atrial flutter with regular atrioventricular (AV) conduction (usually 2:1).

An irregular narrow-complex tachycardia is most likely to be AF, or sometimes atrial flutter with variable block.

Regular narrow-complex tachycardia

Sinus tachycardia
Sinus tachycardia is a common physiological response to stimuli such as exercise or anxiety. In a sick patient it may reflect pain, infection, anaemia, hypovolaemia, or heart failure. Treat the underlying cause.

Paroxysmal supraventricular tachycardia
Atrioventricular nodal re-entry tachycardia is the commonest type of paroxysmal supraventricular tachycardia (SVT), often seen in people without any other form of heart disease. It is uncommon in the peri-arrest setting. It causes a regular, narrow-complex tachycardia, often with no clearly visible atrial activity on the ECG. The heart rate is usually well above the upper limit of normal sinus rate at rest (100 min^{-1}). It is usually benign, unless there is structural heart disease or coronary disease.

Atrioventricular re-entry tachycardia occurs in patients with the WPW syndrome, and is also usually benign, unless there is additional structural heart disease. The common type of AVRT is a regular narrow-complex tachycardia, usually with no visible atrial activity on the ECG.

Atrial flutter
This produces a regular narrow-complex tachycardia. Typical atrial flutter has an atrial rate of about 300 min^{-1}, so atrial flutter with 2:1 conduction produces a tachycardia of about 150 min^{-1} (Figure 13.4). Much faster rates (160 min^{-1} or more) are unlikely to be caused by atrial flutter with 2:1 conduction. Regular tachycardia with slower rates (125–150 min^{-1}) may be caused by atrial flutter with 2:1 conduction, usually when the rate of the atrial flutter has been slowed by drug therapy.

Treatment of regular narrow-complex tachyarrhythmia
If the patient has adverse features and is at risk of deterioration because of the tachyarrhythmia, perform synchronised cardioversion. In this situation it is reasonable to attempt vagal manoeuvres (see below) or to give intravenous adenosine (see below) to a patient with a regular narrow-complex tachyarrhythmia, while preparations are being made for synchronised cardioversion.

In the absence of adverse features:

1 Start with vagal manoeuvres. Carotid sinus massage or the Valsalva manoeuvre will terminate up to a quarter of episodes of paroxysmal SVT. Record an ECG (preferably multi-lead) during each manoeuvre. If the rhythm is atrial flutter with 2:1 conduction, slowing of the ventricular response will often occur and reveal flutter waves (Figure 13.5).
2 If the arrhythmia persists and is not atrial flutter, give adenosine 6 mg as a very rapid intravenous bolus. Use a relatively large cannula and large (e.g. antecubital) vein. Warn the patient that they will feel unwell and probably experience chest discomfort for a few seconds after the injection. Record an ECG during the injection. If the ventricular rate slows transiently, look for atrial activity, such as atrial flutter or other atrial tachycardia, and treat accordingly. If there is no response to adenosine 6 mg, give a 12 mg bolus. If there is no response give one further 12 mg bolus.
3 Vagal manoeuvres or adenosine will terminate almost all AVNRT or AVRT within seconds. Failure to terminate a regular narrow-complex tachycardia with adenosine suggests an atrial tachycardia such as atrial flutter.
4 If adenosine is contraindicated, or fails to terminate a regular narrow-complex tachycardia without demonstrating that it is atrial flutter, consider giving a calcium-channel blocker, for example verapamil 2.5–5.0 mg intravenously over 2 min.

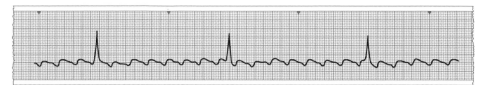

Figure 13.5 Atrial flutter with a high degree of atrioventricular block. Copyright © 2012 Dr Oliver Meyer, Reproduced with permission.

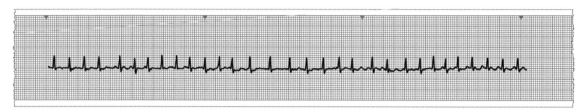

Figure 13.6 Atrial fibrillation. Copyright © 2012 Dr Oliver Meyer, Reproduced with permission.

Irregular narrow-complex tachycardia

An irregular narrow-complex tachycardia is most likely to be AF with a rapid ventricular response (Figure 13.6) or, less commonly, atrial flutter with variable AV conduction.

If the patient has adverse features and is at risk of deterioration because of the tachyarrhythmia, perform synchronised cardioversion. In the absence of contraindications, start anticoagulation – initially with low-molecular-weight heparin or unfractionated heparin (see later) – at the earliest opportunity. Do not allow this treatment to delay cardioversion.

If there are no adverse features, immediate treatment options include:

- Rate control by drug therapy
- Rhythm control using drugs to achieve chemical cardioversion
- Rhythm control by synchronised cardioversion
- Treatment to prevent complications (e.g. anticoagulation)

The longer a patient remains in AF the greater is the likelihood of atrial thrombus developing. In general, patients who have been in AF for more than 48 h should not be treated by cardioversion (electrical or chemical) until they have been fully anticoagulated for at least 3 weeks, or unless transoesophageal echocardiography has detected no evidence of atrial thrombus. If the clinical situation dictates that cardioversion is needed more urgently, give either low-molecular-weight heparin in therapeutic dose or an intravenous bolus injection of unfractionated heparin followed by a continuous infusion to maintain the activated partial thromboplastin time (APTT) at 1.5–2.0 times the reference control value. Continue heparin therapy and commence oral anticoagulation after successful cardioversion. The duration of anticoagulation should be a minimum of 4 weeks, often substantially longer.

If the aim is to control heart rate, the usual drug of choice is a beta-blocker. Diltiazem may be used in patients in whom beta blockade is contraindicated or not tolerated; in the UK, only the oral form of diltiazem is available. Digoxin may be used in patients with heart failure. Amiodarone may be used to assist with rate control but is most useful in maintaining rhythm control. Magnesium is also used but the data supporting this are limited.

If the duration of AF is less than 48 h and rhythm control is considered the appropriate strategy, chemical cardioversion may be appropriate. Seek expert help with the use of drugs such as flecainide. Do not use flecainide in the presence of heart failure, known left ventricular impairment or ischaemic heart disease, or a prolonged QT interval. Amiodarone (300 mg i.v. over 20–60 min followed by 900 mg over 24 h) may be used to attempt chemical cardioversion but is less often effective and takes longer. Electrical cardioversion remains an option in this setting and will restore sinus rhythm in more patients than chemical cardioversion.

Seek expert help if a patient with AF is known or found to have ventricular pre-excitation (WPW syndrome). Avoid using adenosine, diltiazem, verapamil, or digoxin in patients with pre-excited AF or atrial flutter as these drugs block the AV node and may cause a relative increase in pre-excitation.

Bradyarrhythmia

Bradycardia is defined as a resting heart rate of $<60 \, \text{min}^{-1}$. It may be:

- Physiological (e.g. in athletes)
- Cardiac in origin (e.g. atrioventricular block or sinus node disease)
- Non-cardiac in origin (e.g. vasovagal, hypothermia, hypothyroidism, hyperkalaemia)
- Drug-induced (e.g. beta blockade, diltiazem, digoxin, amiodarone)

Assess the patient with bradycardia using the ABCDE approach. Consider the potential cause of the bradycardia, look for adverse signs (Figure 13.7), and treat any reversible causes.

If adverse features are present initial treatment is usually pharmacological; pacing is used for patients in whom initial pharmacological treatment is ineffective or inadequate and those with risk factors for asystole. If there are no adverse features or high risk of progression to asystole, do not initiate immediate treatment, but continue monitoring.

Pharmacological treatment for bradycardia

If adverse features are present, give atropine, 500 microgram i.v. and repeat every 3–5 min, as required, to a total of 3 mg. Doses of

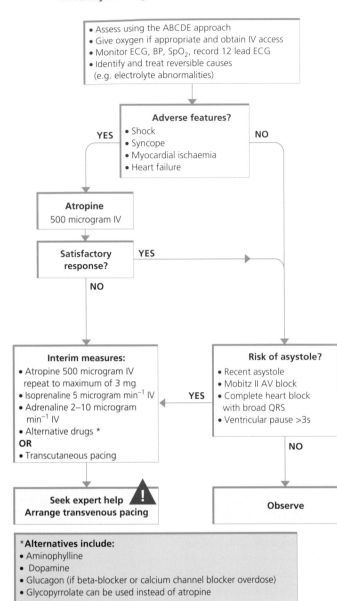

Adult bradycardia algorithm

- Assess using the ABCDE approach
- Give oxygen if appropriate and obtain IV access
- Monitor ECG, BP, SpO₂, record 12 lead ECG
- Identify and treat reversible causes
  (e.g. electrolyte abnormalities)

Adverse features?
- Shock
- Syncope
- Myocardial ischaemia
- Heart failure

YES   NO

Atropine
500 microgram IV

Satisfactory response?   YES

NO

Interim measures:
- Atropine 500 microgram IV repeat to maximum of 3 mg
- Isoprenaline 5 microgram min⁻¹ IV
- Adrenaline 2–10 microgram min⁻¹ IV
- Alternative drugs *
OR
- Transcutaneous pacing

Risk of asystole?
- Recent asystole
- Mobitz II AV block
- Complete heart block with broad QRS
- Ventricular pause >3s

YES

NO

Seek expert help
Arrange transvenous pacing

Observe

*Alternatives include:
- Aminophylline
- Dopamine
- Glucagon (if beta-blocker or calcium channel blocker overdose)
- Glycopyrrolate can be used instead of atropine

Figure 13.7 The adult bradycardia algorithm. Reproduced with the kind permission of the Resuscitation Council (UK).

atropine of <500 microgram can cause paradoxical slowing of the heart rate.

If bradycardia with adverse signs persists despite atropine, consider cardiac pacing. If pacing cannot be achieved promptly, consider the use of second-line drugs.

In some clinical settings second-line drugs may be appropriate before the use of cardiac pacing. For example, consider giving intravenous glucagon if a beta-blocker or calcium channel blocker is a likely cause of the bradycardia. Consider using digoxin-specific antibody fragments for bradycardia caused by digoxin toxicity.

Consider using theophylline (100–200 mg by slow intravenous injection) for bradycardia complicating acute inferior wall myocardial infarction, spinal cord injury or cardiac transplantation. Do not give atropine to patients with cardiac transplants. The denervated heart will not respond to vagal blockade by atropine, which may cause paradoxical sinus arrest or high-grade AV block. Other options for second-line drug therapy include infusion of isoprenaline (5 microgram min⁻¹ starting dose), adrenaline (2–10 microgram min⁻¹), or dopamine (2.5–10 microgram kg⁻¹ min⁻¹).

Cardiac pacing for bradycardia

Initiate transcutaneous pacing immediately (see Chapter 14) in a patient with bradycardia and adverse features if there is no response to atropine or if atropine is unlikely to be effective.

Transcutaneous pacing can be painful and may fail to achieve effective electrical 'capture' (i.e. a QRS complex after the pacing stimulus) or fail to achieve a mechanical response (i.e. palpable pulse). Verify electrical capture on the monitor or ECG and check that it is producing a pulse. Reassess the patient's condition. Use analgesia and sedation as necessary to control pain and attempt to identify the cause of the bradyarrhythmia.

Seek expert help to assess the need for temporary transvenous pacing and to initiate this when appropriate. Consider temporary transvenous pacing if there is documented recent asystole (ventricular standstill of >3 s), Mobitz type II AV block, or complete (third-degree) AV block (especially with broad QRS or initial heart rate <40 min⁻¹).

Acknowledgement

The text of this chapter has been adapted with permission from *Advanced Life Support* 6th edition, London, Resuscitation Council (UK), 2011.

Further reading

Blomstrom-Lundqvist C, Scheinmann MM. ACC/AHA/ESC guidelines for the management of patients with supraventricular arrhythmias. Executive Summary. *Eur Heart J* 2003;**24**:1857–97. See also www.escardio.org.

European Heart Rhythm Association, European Association for Cardio-thoracic Surgery, Camm AJ *et al.* Guidelines for the management of atrial fibrillation: the Task Force for the Management of Atrial Fibrillation of the European Society of Cardiology (ESC). *Eur Heart J* 2010;**31**:2369–429. See also www.escardio.org.

Vardas PE, Auricchio A, Blanc JJ, *et al.* ESC Guidelines for cardiac pacing and cardiac resynchronization therapy: The Task Force for Cardiac Pacing and Cardiac Resynchronization Therapy of the European Society of Cardiology. Developed in collaboration with the European Heart Rhythm Association. *Eur Heart J* 2007;**28**:2256–95. See also www.escardio.org.

Zipes DP, Camm AJ. ACC/AHA/ESC 2006 guidelines for management of patients with ventricular arrhythmias and the prevention of sudden death. Executive Summary. *Eur Heart J* 2006;**27**:2099–140. See also www.escardio.org.

CHAPTER 14

Pacemakers and Implantable Cardioverter-Defibrillators

Rani Robson[1] and Jerry Nolan[2]

[1]British Heart Institute, Bristol, UK
[2]Royal United Hospital, Bath, UK

OVERVIEW

- Temporary pacing techniques include percussion pacing, transcutaneous pacing and transvenous pacing. These are emergency measures, which are used until either resolution of the bradycardia or definitive invasive pacing has been established
- Permanent pacemakers are used to treat severe bradycardia, to promote cardiac resynchronisation and as implantable cardioverter-defibrillators for the treatment of life-threatening ventricular arrhythmias

---

Introduction

Cardiac pacing devices can be either temporary or permanent. Temporary techniques include percussion (fist) pacing, transcutaneous pacing and transvenous pacing. Permanent pacemakers (PPM) are used for the treatment of severe bradycardia, and for left ventricular pacing as part of cardiac resynchronisation therapy (CRT) for the treatment of chronic heart failure; implantable cardioverter-defibrillators (ICDs) are used for the treatment of life-threatening ventricular arrhythmias.

Understanding the methods for providing temporary pacing is invaluable in resuscitation care. With the increased prevalence of pacemakers and ICDs, an awareness of the capabilities and complications associated with devices is essential.

Indications for pacing and ICDs

An abbreviated summary of indications adapted from the ACC/AHA/HRS 2008 and NICE 2007 guidelines are shown in Box 14.1.

Methods of pacing

Non-invasive pacing

Both percussion pacing and transcutaneous pacing can be used to treat profound bradycardia causing severe haemodynamic instability or cardiac arrest. Non-invasive pacing is an emergency measure

used until either resolution of the bradycardia or definitive invasive pacing has been established.

Box 14.1 **Indications for pacing and ICDs**

Indications for emergency pacing
Any bradycardia causing:

> Syncope at rest
> Haemodynamic compromise
> Bradycardia induced ventricular tachyarrhythmias

NB: If a permanent pacemaker is indicated, avoid temporary pacing and arrange for urgent implantation of a permanent system

Indications for permanent pacing (PPM)
Definite indications:

> Symptomatic 3rd degree or 2nd degree heart block
> Sustained VT caused by pauses
> Bifascicular block with intermittent 3rd degree or 2nd degree, or alternating bundle branch block
> Trifascicular block with intermittent 3rd degree or 2nd degree block
> Sinus bradycardia and pauses causing symptoms
> Symptomatic chronotropic incompetence
> Symptomatic bradycardia resulting from essential medications
> Carotid sinus hypersensitivity resulting in syncope caused by pauses of >3 s
> 3rd degree or 2nd degree (Type II) heart block in AF with pauses of ≥5 s

Relative indications:

> Asymptomatic 3rd degree or 2nd degree (Type II) heart block
> Sinus bradycardia of <40 during waking hours
> Syncope of unexplained origin where EP study demonstrates sinus node disease
> Syncope with bifascicular block where other causes have been excluded
> Significantly symptomatic neurocardiogenic syncope associated with bradycardia

Indications for cardiac resynchronisation therapy (CRT)
Definite indications (patient with all of the following):

> Sinus rhythm
> Ejection Fraction (EF) of ≤35%
> QRS ≥0.12 s

ABC of Resuscitation, Sixth Edition. Edited by Jasmeet Soar, Gavin D. Perkins and Jerry Nolan.
© 2013 John Wiley & Sons, Ltd. Published 2013 by John Wiley & Sons, Ltd.

On optimal medical therapy
Class III or IV NYHA symptoms

Relative indications (patients fulfilling all of the criteria for definite indications but have the following):

Atrial fibrillation
QRS <0.12 s, but requiring a high burden of RV pacing

Indications for implantable cardioverter defibrillator (ICD)
Secondary prevention:

Patients (in the absence of a treatable cause) presenting with either
Cardiac arrest caused by VT or VF
Spontaneous VT causing syncope or haemodynamic compromise
Sustained VT with EF <35%

Primary prevention:

Patients with a history of myocardial infarction (>4 weeks previously) and either:
EF <35%, non-sustained VT (NSVT) on Holter and VT at electrophysiological testing
EF <30% and QRS >120 ms
Familial cardiac condition with a high risk of sudden death

Percussion pacing

When bradycardia is so profound that it causes clinical cardiac arrest, percussion pacing may produce an adequate cardiac output and negate the need for CPR. It enables either recovery of a spontaneous cardiac rhythm or maintenance of vital organ perfusion before implementation of transcutaneous or transvenous pacing. Percussion pacing is more likely to be successful when ventricular standstill is accompanied by continuing P wave activity. Percussion pacing is not as reliable as electrical pacing; if it fails, start CPR immediately. See Box 14.2 for an outline of how to perform percussion pacing.

Box 14.2 How to perform percussion pacing

- With the side of a closed fist raised about 10 cm above the chest, deliver repeated firm blows to the precordium lateral to the lower left sternal edge
- If these do not generate QRS complexes, try using slightly harder blows and move the point of contact around the precordium until a site is found that produces repeated ventricular stimulation

---

Transcutaneous pacing

Compared with transvenous pacing, non-invasive transcutaneous pacing is simpler and quicker to implement (Box 14.3).

Box 14.3 How to perform transcutaneous pacing

- Attach ECG monitoring electrodes and leads if necessary – these are needed with some transcutaneous pacing devices

---

- Position the electrode pads in either the conventional right pectoral-apical (preferred) or the anterior-posterior (A-P) positions (Figure 14.1)
- If using a pacing device that is not capable of defibrillation, use A-P positions for the pacing electrodes so that defibrillator pads can still be used in the right pectoral and apical positions if cardiac arrest occurs
- Most transcutaneous pacing devices offer pacing in demand mode; the pacemaker will be inhibited if it detects a spontaneous QRS complex. Beware of movement artefact, which may also inhibit the pacemaker and may necessitate switching to fixed-rate pacing mode
- Select an appropriate pacing rate. This will usually be in the range of 60–90 min^{-1} for adults, but in some circumstances (for example complete AV block with an idioventricular rhythm at 50 min^{-1}) a slower pacing rate of 40 or even 30 min^{-1} may be appropriate to deliver pacing only during sudden ventricular standstill or more extreme bradycardia
- If the pacing device has an adjustable energy output set this at its lowest value and turn on the pacemaker. Gradually increase the output while observing the patient and the ECG. As the current is increased the muscles of the chest wall will contract with each impulse and a pacing spike will appear on the ECG. Increase the current until each pacing spike is followed immediately by a QRS complex, which indicates electrical capture (Figure 14.2) (typically with a current of 50–100 mA using a device with adjustable output)
- Check that the apparent QRS complex is followed by a T wave. Occasionally, artefact generated by the pacing current travelling through the chest may be mistaken for a QRS complex; this artefact will not be followed by a T wave
- If the highest current setting is reached and electrical capture has not occurred, try changing the electrode positions. Continued failure to achieve electrical capture may indicate non-viable myocardium
- Having achieved electrical capture with the pacemaker, check for a pulse, which confirms 'mechanical capture' of the ventricle. Absence of a pulse in the presence of good electrical capture constitutes pulseless electrical activity (PEA).

Conscious patients usually experience considerable discomfort during transcutaneous pacing and will often require intravenous analgesia and/or sedation. When defibrillating a patient who has pacing-only electrode pads in place, apply the defibrillator paddles at least 2–3 cm from the pacing electrodes to prevent arcing of the defibrillation current. Chest compressions can be given and other manual contact with the patient maintained as necessary with transcutaneous electrodes in place. When transcutaneous pacing produces an adequate cardiac output seek expert help immediately to insert a transvenous pacing lead.

Invasive pacing
Temporary transvenous pacing

Temporary transvenous pacing (Figure 14.3) carries the risk of significant complications and should be undertaken independently only by experienced practitioners. Under sterile conditions and

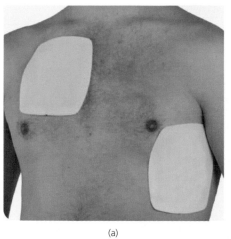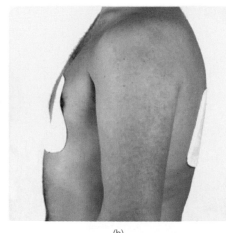

(a)　　　　　　　　　　　　　　(b)

Figure 14.1 Transcutaneous pacing using electrode pads in the (a) conventional right pectoral-apical or (b) anterior-posterior (A-P) positions. Photograph reproduced with kind permission by Michael Scott and the Resuscitation Council (UK).

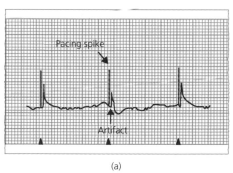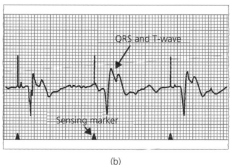

(a)　　　　　　　　　　　　　　(b)

Figure 14.2 Transcutaneous pacing ECG showing (a) pacing spike and artefact, and (b) pacing spike followed by ventricular capture. Copyright © 2012 Dr Oliver Meyer, Reproduced with permission.

using radiographic screening, a pacing wire is inserted into either the femoral, right internal jugular or right subclavian vein and the tip positioned at the apex of the right ventricle. Some slack should be left in the wire to allow for cardiac movement in deep inspiration and firmly secured to the skin to avoid dislodgement.

The basic requirements for effective temporary transvenous pacing include the following:

- Ideally, the pacing threshold should be <1 V. If an alternative stable position cannot be achieved, a threshold of 1.5 V may be tolerated
- Using the demand mode, set the device output to 3 V or 3 times higher than the threshold
- In complete heart block or severe bradycardia, set the rate at 70–80 min^{-1}. Where the base rate is reasonable and the pacing is being used for pauses, the rate is set just below the intrinsic rate. Where pacing is being used to prevent ventricular ectopics resulting in ventricular arrhythmias, the rate is set at 80–90 min^{-1}

Permanent transvenous pacing

Permanent pacemaker generators are usually positioned below the clavicle, between the subcutaneous tissue and the pectoral muscle. The generator may be placed underneath the pectoral muscle in particularly thin patients or those with previous wound complications. The leads will be positioned under radiographic screening, either via the brachiocephalic, subclavian or axillary veins (Figure 14.4).

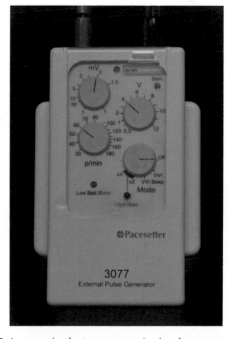

Figure 14.3 An example of a temporary pacing box for transvenous pacing.

Epicardial and subcutaneous leads

Epicardial leads are surgically placed on the external surface of the heart. They are used routinely as a prophylactic temporary measure after aortic valve surgery. Subcutaneous leads with shocking coils

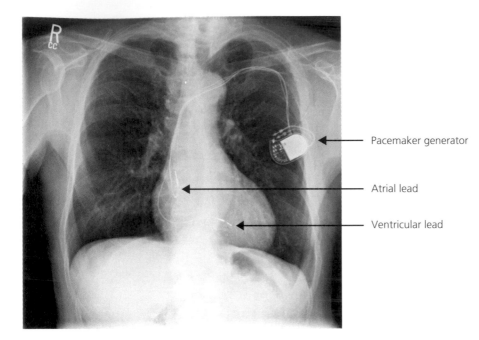

Figure 14.4 Chest radiograph showing a dual chamber permanent pacemaker.

are used occasionally in patients requiring an ICD who have a high defibrillation threshold or in whom transvenous lead positioning is best avoided.

Concepts in pacing and internal cardiac defibrillation

Pace threshold

An artificial pacemaker generates an electrical pacing stimulus that excites cardiac tissue resulting in a wave front of action potentials propagating away from the stimulus. The minimum stimulus intensity and duration necessary to reliably result in myocardial capture is known as the pacing threshold. The pacing threshold will be affected by the integrity of the contact between the electrode and the myocardium and the electrical property of the myocardial tissue being paced (potentially altered by drugs, ischaemia, electrolyte imbalance).

Pacing mode

There is a three-letter international code that describes the basic pacemaker function. The first letter refers to the chamber paced, the second to the chamber sensed and the third to how the device responds to a sensed event (Table 14.1). Often a fourth letter is used to describe additional features (Table 14.2) such as rate response (R) – an accelerometer within the device detects the patient's physical activity and varies the pacing rate accordingly.

Table 14.1 International pacing code.

Chamber paced	Chamber sensed	Response to sensed event
V – ventricle	V – ventricle	I – inhibits
A – atrium	A – atrium	T – triggers
D – Dual (both A&V)	D – dual (both A&V)	D – dual (I&T)

Table 14.2 Common pacing modes.

VVI(±R)	The ventricle is paced, the ventricle is sensed and the device is inhibited following a sensed event
DDD(±R)	Both chambers are paced, both chambers are sensed and the device will respond by either inhibiting or triggering a paced event depending on the chamber sensed
VDD(±R)	The ventricle is paced, both chambers are sensed and ventricular pacing is either triggered or inhibited depending on which chamber is sensed

The magnet mode

Pacemakers and ICDs are potentially susceptible to electromagnetic interference such as that caused by diathermy, radio-frequency ablation and therapeutic ionising radiation. Pacemakers and ICDs switch to magnet mode when sufficiently close to a strong magnetic field. With a pacemaker, the magnet mode will be a non-sensing fixed pacing mode at a predetermined rate (usually 70–80 beats per minute); with an ICD, the magnet mode will disarm all therapies and the ICD will deliver only pacing at the programmed rate. When using diathermy, there is a risk that the pacemaker will sense the electromagnetic interference and inhibit pacing. An ICD may detect the electromagnetic interference as ventricular fibrillation (VF). By applying a magnet to the skin over a pacemaker generator, sensing will be switched off and pacing will occur.

Most pacemaker devices and all ICDs are incompatible with MRI – strong magnetic fields can cause significant malfunction of the device. Some newer permanent pacemaker models are compatible with MRI scanning.

Any device that has been affected by a magnet must be checked formally using the device programmer.

Implantable cardioverter defibrillators

The shocking electrodes of an ICD are specialised, high-surface-area coils along the length of the right ventricular (RV) lead that deliver energy rapidly to the heart muscle. Using complex sensing algorithms, the ICD differentiates between pathological life-threatening ventricular arrhythmias and atrial arrhythmias or sinus tachycardia.

Ventricular tachycardia (VT) may be terminated with a burst of paced beats (usually 6–12) at a rate faster than the VT circuit. This is known as anti-tachycardia pacing (ATP); it carries a 1–5% risk of accelerating VT into VF. If ATP fails to terminate the VT, the device will give a defibrillatory shock.

Currently, most ICDs deliver energy of up to 41 J biphasic via the shocking coil. For VF, or VT faster than a predetermined rate, a defibrillatory shock will be delivered from the outset. The device will deliver a programmed number of shocks. On subsequent attempts at defibrillation, the shock vector (direction) may be altered according to the device programming. Once the device has delivered all programmed shocks, therapy is discontinued even if the patient remains in VT or VF.

Troubleshooting devices

Patients with pacemakers or ICDs are routinely seen in device follow-up clinics: the lead threshold, sensitivity and impedance are checked and the programming and battery life assessed.

Failure to pace

The pacemaker will fail to pace if the capture threshold exceeds the device output. See Box 14.4 for a list of causes of high pacing threshold.

Box 14.4 Causes of high pacing threshold

- Lead displacement
- Lead fracture: a pacing spike may still be seen on the surface ECG but it is not transmitted to the lead tip; lead impedance will be very high. A common cause of lead fracture is crush as the lead passes between the clavicle and the first rib
- A break in the lead insulation: if the inner lead remains intact then pacing may continue but the battery will be rapidly depleted; lead impedance will be low
- Exit block: the pacing stimulus fails to propagate beyond the tip of the lead. This may be due to a fibrous cap over the tip of the lead, myocardial ischaemia, electrolyte abnormalities or drugs (such as flecainide).

Over-sensing of artefact (e.g. from muscle activity) may result in failure to pace. All ICDs have the capacity to pace a bradycardia, but many patients with an ICD have no indication for bradycardia pacing. An ICD may be programmed to pace only in the context of a bradycardia of less than 40 beats per minute.

Failure to deliver appropriate ICD therapy

Failure to deliver appropriate ICD therapy (Box 14.5) can be fatal.

Box 14.5 Causes of failure to deliver appropriate ICD therapy

- The therapies on the ICD have been switched off (such as during surgery when using diathermy)
- The rate of the VT is slower then the ICD programmed minimum detection rate for VT therapy. Drugs such as amiodarone may slow VT rate
- The ICD under-senses the VT or the VT is inappropriately discriminated as an SVT

Use external defibrillation if an ICD is failing to deliver therapy in compromised VT or VF. This is done safely by applying a device magnet to disarm ICD therapies, positioning the defibrillation pads in the antero-lateral positions (ideally with the pads >8 cm from the generator) and following ALS defibrillation guidelines. If the patient has a right-sided ICD generator (rare), apply the pads in the antero-posterior position.

Failure of therapy to terminate VT or VF

An ICD may fail to terminate VT or VF if the defibrillation threshold is too high. This may occur in the presence of severely dilated left ventricles, cardiac ischaemia or electrolyte abnormalities. Correct reversible causes of a high defibrillation threshold. If the VT or VF temporarily terminates and then restarts, the device will deliver therapies from the beginning of programming; thus, a patient with recurrent VT or VF may receive many therapies. Treat the cause of recurrent VT/VF and give appropriate antiarrhythmic drugs. If necessary, disarm the ICD with a magnet.

Inappropriate ICD therapy

Inappropriate ICD therapy may be delivered if sinus tachycardia, supraventricular tachycardia (SVT) is detected incorrectly as VF/VT or if there is interference. In an emergency, placing a device magnet over the ICD generator will disarm ICD therapies.

Tracking of atrial arrhythmias

In dual chamber sensing devices, atrial tachycardias such as atrial flutter or atrial arrhythmias can result in rapid ventricular pacing if the atrial rate falls within the rate settings of the device. Ventricular tracking of atrial arrhythmias can be overcome by programming the device to mode switch under such conditions to VVI or DDI. The atrial arrhythmia should be treated.

Further reading

ACC/AHA/HRS 2008 Guidelines for device-based therapy of cardiac rhythm abnormalities *J Am Coll Cardiol* 2008;**51**;2085–105.
Implantable Cardioverter Defibrillators, review of technology appraisal 11. NICE, July 2007.

CHAPTER 15

Cardiorespiratory Arrest in Advanced Pregnancy

David A. Gabbott

Gloucester Royal Hospital, Gloucester, UK

OVERVIEW

- Maternal cardiorespiratory arrest is rare and often preceded by maternal collapse
- The physiological changes in advanced pregnancy may require modification of the ABC approach to cardiopulmonary resuscitation (CPR)
- Avoid aortocaval compression and the reduction in maternal cardiac output this causes; however, do not compromise quality of chest compressions delivered
- Undertake perimortem Caesarean section within 5 minutes of maternal cardiac arrest if no return of spontaneous circulation
- The use of Obstetric Early Warning Systems and greater emphasis on recognition and training should improve survival

Introduction

Maternal cardiorespiratory arrest is fortunately an infrequent yet catastrophic event. Triennial audits from the UK have repeatedly confirmed that major haemorrhage, thromboembolism, amniotic fluid embolism and hypertensive disease of pregnancy (PET and eclampsia) account for the majority of 'direct' obstetric related deaths. Data from the latest Centre for Maternal and Child Enquiry (CMACE) triennial report (2011) indicate a maternal mortality rate in the UK of 14/100,000; sepsis is now an additional leading 'direct' cause of death. Cardiac disease continues to be the leading 'indirect' cause of death, which is attributed to the increased prevalence of lifestyle risk factors (obesity, smoking and increased maternal age), peripartum cardiomyopathy, aortic dissection and the increased number of women surviving and becoming pregnant with pre-existing complex congenital heart disease.

Maternal collapse (which may or may not lead to cardiorespiratory arrest) occurs in 3–6 mothers per 1000 pregnancies. Major haemorrhage is overwhelmingly the most likely cause and increasingly better recognition and management has significantly reduced mortality in this situation.

Whether maternal collapse or cardiorespiratory arrest, this is a stressful and emotive situation in which there are potentially two lives that may be lost. The best hope for fetal survival is maternal survival.

Physiological changes

The physiological changes that occur during advanced pregnancy may alter management of cardiorespiratory arrest in the parturient: the ABC approach requires some modifications.

Airway

Laryngeal and tracheal oedema is more prevalent in advanced pregnancy and the pharyngeal mucosa is hyperaemic and more friable. The cross-sectional area of the upper airway is narrower in pregnancy. There is an increasing risk of aspiration from progesterone-induced gastro-oesophageal reflux and use of cricoid pressure may be necessary. Difficulty with tracheal intubation is more common in late pregnancy. Some of the standard indicators of a potentially difficult airway (e.g. short thyromental distance and poor jaw slide) may improve as pregnancy advances; thus, these surrogate markers are unreliable for predicting difficult tracheal intubation. The difficulties associated with tracheal intubation may also relate to:

- Large breasts
- Full dentition
- Glottic oedema
- Poorly applied cricoid pressure

Potentially difficult tracheal intubation and the threat of aspiration are reasons for the individual who is not skilled in tracheal intubation to use a supraglottic airway device with a gastric drain port for airway control during CPR. Such devices include the LMA Supreme and the igel airway (Figures 15.1 and 15.2).

Breathing

The gravid uterus displaces the diaphragm causing a decrease in functional residual capacity (FRC) and decrease in chest wall compliance. This makes ventilation of the lungs more difficult and may necessitate higher inflation pressures during positive pressure ventilation – optimal bag-mask ventilation is impaired. Intrapulmonary shunting increases in pregnancy (up to 15%) and together with the increased oxygen requirements during advanced pregnancy, contributes to rapidly developing hypoxia during apnoea.

ABC of Resuscitation, Sixth Edition. Edited by Jasmeet Soar, Gavin D. Perkins and Jerry Nolan.
© 2013 John Wiley & Sons, Ltd. Published 2013 by John Wiley & Sons, Ltd.

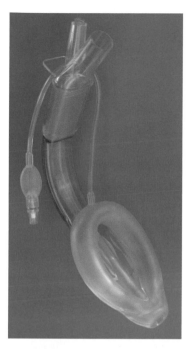

Figure 15.1 Supreme LMA.

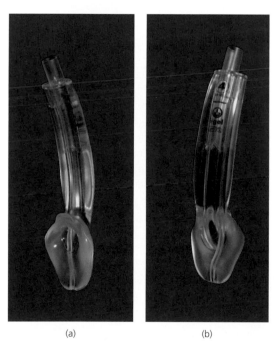

(a)   (b)

Figure 15.2 I-gel airway.

Maternal arterial carbon dioxide values are lower than normal because of hyperventilation caused by a progesterone-driven increase in tidal volume and minute ventilation. This may reduce the buffering capacity of the plasma and makes the development of an acidosis more likely in the setting of cardiorespiratory arrest.

Circulation

Plasma volume is increased in the parturient and there is a physiological or dilutional anaemia. This reduces oxygen carrying capacity.

The heart rate increases and cardiac output may be up to 50% greater in the advanced stages of pregnancy. There is a decrease in systemic vascular resistance, which lowers systolic blood pressure. Uterine blood flow may be as much as 12% of cardiac output and this increases the risk of massive haemorrhage from this source.

The circulatory adjustments during CPR focus on avoidance of aortocaval compression. This phenomenon reduces both blood supply to the uterus (and therefore fetus) and, more importantly, maternal venous return to the heart. Cardiac output may be reduced by up to 35–40% in the supine parturient. Furthermore, maternal cardiac output may be persistently impaired despite efforts to reduce compression of the inferior vena cava (IVC) until delivery of the foetus. The risk for IVC compression is greater as pregnancy progresses and begins to occur as the uterus becomes visible above the pelvis. The problem is compounded by multiple pregnancy and conditions that cause pathological uterine enlargement (e.g. polyhydramnios).

Table 15.1 shows the physiological changes in advanced pregnancy and the potential effect on CPR.

Cardiopulmonary resuscitation guidelines 2010

The 2010 resuscitation guidelines for adults are followed with a few modifications for maternal resuscitation. Standard drug doses, defibrillation energies and compression ventilation ratios are used.

Drugs

The dose of adrenaline for all cardiac arrests and the dose of amiodarone for shock resistant ventricular fibrillation remain 1 mg and 300 mg respectively. Fibrinolytic drugs are recommended for massive pulmonary embolism although subsequent Caesarean section will be challenging. The potential effects on the fetus should not preclude their use during cardiac arrest.

The gravid uterus may reduce venous return – deliver drugs via a route that avoids the IVC, such as the upper limb. If venous access is difficult, insert an intra-osseous needle in the upper humerus.

Defibrillation

Transthoracic impedance in pregnancy is the same as the non-pregnant state; the same defibrillation energies are used. Delivery of an electric shock across the maternal chest does not harm the fetus. Current travelling directly through the uterus, for example electrocution from domestic electricity, may injure the fetus. Use of self-adhesive, multifunction electrodes/pads eliminates placement problems associated with large breasts and lateral tilt.

Chest compression

The 2010 guidelines emphasise improvement of the quality of chest compressions by increasing both the depth (5–6 cm) and frequency (100–120 per minute), ensuring adequate chest wall recoil and minimises interruption to chest compressions. Aortocaval compression must be avoided during CPR in advanced pregnancy. Although manikin studies have demonstrated that it is possible to perform

Table 15.1 Physiological changes in advanced pregnancy and the potential effect on CPR.

	Change in pregnancy	Potential impact during CPR
Cardiovascular system		
Plasma volume	Increased by up to 50%	Dilutional anaemia Reduced oxygen carrying capacity
Heart rate	Increased by up to 30%	Increased oxygen and CPR demand
Cardiac output	Increased by up to 50%	Increased oxygen and CPR demand
Systemic vascular resistance	Decreased by up to 40%	Reduced coronary and cerebral perfusion during CPR
Venous return	Decreased by pressure of gravid uterus on IVC	Significant reduction in cardiac output generated by CPR
Uterine blood flow	Up to 12% of cardiac output	Potential for rapid and massive haemorrhage
Respiratory system		
Tidal volume and minute ventilation	Increased by up to 45%	Hyperventilation reduces arterial PCO_2 and plasma HCO_3 Reduced buffering capacity
Oxygen consumption	Increased by up to 30%	Rapid development of hypoxia
Functional Residual Capacity	Decreased by up to 25% by pressure of gravid uterus	Increased intrapulmonary shunting.
Chest wall compliance	Reduced	Higher airway pressures Difficulty with ventilation
Pharynx	Hyperaemic	Airway narrowing Difficult tracheal intubation Bleeding if damaged
Larynx	Hyperaemic and oedema	Airway narrowing Difficult tracheal intubation
Other changes		
Gastric motility	Reduced	Increased risk of aspiration
Lower oesophageal sphincter	Relaxed	Increased risk of aspiration
Uterus	Enlarged Up to 10% of cardiac output	Reduction in venous return from IVC compression Diaphragm splinting reduces lung compliance and increases intrapulmonary shunting Potential for massive haemorrhage
Weight	Increased	Transfer more difficult Increased breast size may impair ventilation, interfere with tracheal intubation and make positioning of defibrillator pads more difficult

CPR, cardiopulmonary resuscitation; IVC, inferior vena cava.

chest compressions with a patient laterally tilted at various angles, in comparison with the supine position the maximum compression force achieved is reduced significantly. Therefore chest compressions are performed initially with the mother fully supine and the uterus manually displaced laterally. This relieves aortocaval compression while enabling excellent quality chest compressions (Figures 15.3 and 15.4).

Use lateral tilt if it can be achieved without compromising chest compression quality (e.g. on an operating table). Chest compression should generally be performed with the hands in the centre of the chest although the hand position may be slightly higher than normal to adjust for the elevation of the diaphragm and abdominal contents in advanced pregnancy.

Perimortem caesarean section

When initial cardiopulmonary resuscitation attempts fail, delivery of the foetus may improve the chances of successful resuscitation

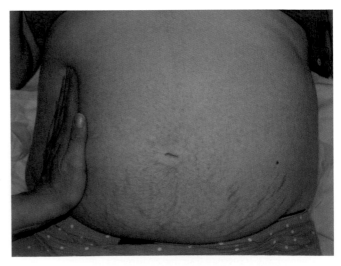

Figure 15.3 Lateral displacement of the uterus using one hand.

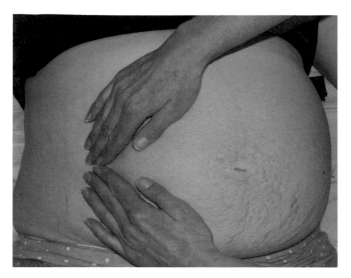

Figure 15.4 Lateral displacement of the uterus using two hands.

of the mother (Figure 15.5). The primary reason for removing the fetus from a gravid uterus is to rapidly restore maternal cardiac output – any benefit to the fetus is secondary. A perimortem Caesarean section will enable access to the abdominal cavity, aortic compression/clamping and use of direct cardiac massage/compression. A perimortem Caesarean section tray should be available on the resuscitation trolley in all areas where maternal collapse may occur, including the emergency department. If immediately available, the use of ultrasound in skilled hands can:

- Rapidly determine the presence of maternal cardiac output
- Determine fetal viability
- Detect the presence of twins
- Localise the placenta prior to opening the abdomen
- Detect concealed uterine haemorrhage

Assessments of fetal viability should not delay the process of perimortem Caesarean section and the gravid uterus should be evacuated even if the foetus is dead.

Timing

Perimortem Caesarean section should be performed when maternal cardiac output has not been restored within 5 minutes. If the gestational age of the mother is 20 weeks or less (uterus has not reached the umbilicus) then the fetus is not viable and compromise to maternal cardiac output is unlikely. Beyond 20 weeks gestation, maternal venous return is compromised and emergency Caesarean section should be performed. After 23 weeks, fetal viability is considered, but this is not the prime reason for evacuating the uterine contents. Fetal outcome improves significantly with gestational age greater than 36 weeks; location of the Caesarean section also influences survival. In the 2011 CMACE report, the highest number of surviving live births after perimortem Caesarean section was achieved in the delivery suite or operating room (7 out of 10). Only one out of 17 neonates survived the procedure in the emergency department. Although most mothers and babies who survive do so when a Caesarean section is performed within 5 minutes, survival of the fetus after longer periods of maternal cardic arrest is well described.

Post-cardiac arrest care

Limited data (case reports) suggest that hypothermia can be used safely in early pregnancy after cardiac arrest if Caesarean section has not been performed. Monitor the fetal heart to enable detection of bradycardia.

Maternal collapse

Recent data from Scotland and Ireland confirm major haemorrhage as the most common cause of maternal morbidity and collapse. Haemorrhage can occur both antenatally and postnatally. Postnatal

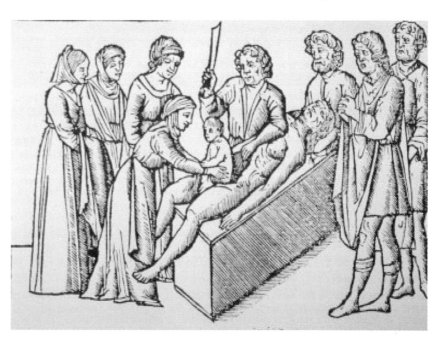

Figure 15.5 A live infant being surgically removed from a dead woman. From Suetonius *Lives of the Twelve Caesars*, 1506.

causes are largely uterine atony and genital tract trauma. Antenatal causes include:

- Ectopic pregnancy
- Uterine rupture
- Placental abruption
- Placenta praevia

A morbidly adherent placenta praevia overlying a previous Caesarean section scar is a major risk. The placenta may be described as 'accreta', 'increta' or 'percreta' depending on the degree of invasion into and beyond the uterine wall. Catastrophic bleeding can be anticipated in these circumstances and all maternity units should have in place a massive haemorrhage protocol for such events. Figure 15.6 shows abnormal placentation.

Techniques for haemorrhage control, both physical and pharmacological, will often be necessary in addition to predicting those mothers at greatest risk, e.g. placenta percreta overlying a previous Caesarean section scar. Oxytocin, carbetocin, ergometrine and prostaglandins (e.g. misoprostol and carboprost) are used for enhancing uterine contraction. Uterine compression sutures, intra-uterine balloons and the use of intravascularly placed catheters/balloons may all reduce uterine haemorrhage considerably. Rapid transfusion systems and cell savers are in common use (Figure 15.7). Fears surrounding amniotic fluid contamination during cell salvage have largely disappeared with the use of more modern filtration techniques. Antifibrinolytic drugs (e.g. tranexamic acid) and early use of blood products, including recombinant Factor VII, are important strategies for treating massive maternal haemorrhage.

Other rare causes of maternal collapse and cardiopulmonary arrest

Drug toxicity

Magnesium is used to treat and prevent eclamptic seizures in pregnancy. Excessive doses may cause:

- Hypotension from vasodilatation
- Reduced muscle power because of its effect at the neuromuscular junction
- Uterine relaxation causing bleeding
- Reduced respiratory rate
- Absent deep tendon reflexes
- ECG changes, e.g. prolonged P–R interval, wide QRS complex, conduction defects
- Cardiac and respiratory arrest

Following cardiac arrest in this setting, use of calcium as a physiological antagonist of magnesium may be life saving.

Epidural bupivacaine is used widely to provide pain relief in labour. Inadvertent intravascular infusion may lead to a sudden loss of consciousness, convulsions and cardiovascular collapse associated with:

- Sinus bradycardia
- Conduction blocks
- Ventricular tachyarrhythmias
- Asystole

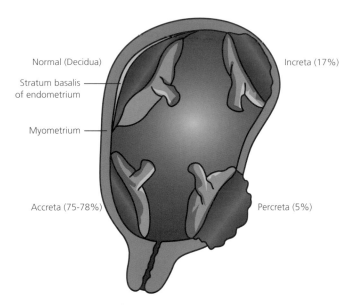

Figure 15.6 Abnormal placentation.

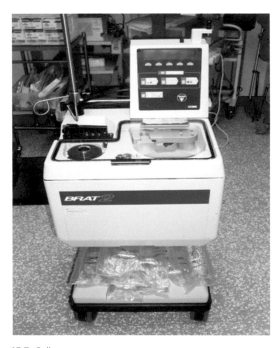

Figure 15.7 Cell saver.

If cardiac arrest is associated with local anaesthetic toxicity, intralipid is given and prolonged CPR may be required (Figure 15.8). The mechanism of action of lipid remains uncertain but it may involve extraction of lipophilic bupivacaine from aqueous plasma/tissues or the counteraction of bupivacaine inhibition of myocardial fatty acid oxidation.

Maternal Early Warning Systems (MEWS)

The recently published document 'Providing equity of critical and maternity care for the critically ill pregnant or recently pregnant woman' (2011) has stated that all maternity services should implement the NICE guideline on the 'Care of the Critically Ill in

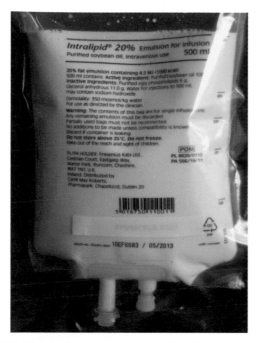

Figure 15.8 Lipid emulsion for the treatment of cardiac arrest associated with local anaesthetic.

Hospital'. Physiological track and trigger systems should be used to monitor all antenatal and postnatal admissions. A graded response strategy for patients identified as being at risk of clinical deterioration should be agreed and delivered locally. It is anticipated that a National Maternal Early Warning System will be developed. Greater emphasis on recognising the sick mother and training those who may only rarely encounter cardiorespiratory arrest in the parturient should improve survival.

Further reading

Ahearn G, Hadjiliadis D, Govert J, Tapson V. Massive pulmonary embolism during pregnancy successfully treated with recombinant tissue plasminogen activator. *Arch Int Med* 2002;**162**:1221–7.

Centre for Maternal and Child Enquiries (CMACE). Saving Mothers' Lives: reviewing maternal deaths to make motherhood safer: 2006–08. The Eighth Report on Confidential Enquiries into Maternal Deaths in the United Kingdom. *BJOG* 2011;**118**(Suppl. 1):1–203.

Deakin CD, Morrison LJ, Morley PT, et al. Part 8: Advanced life support: 2010 International Consensus on Cardiopulmonary Resuscitation and Emergency Cardiovascular Care Science with Treatment Recommendations. *Resuscitation* 2010;**81**(Suppl 1):e93–e174.

Deakin CD, Nolan JP, Soar J, *et al.* European Resuscitation Council Guidelines for Resuscitation 2010 Section 4. Adult advanced life support. *Resuscitation* 2010;**81**:1305–52.

Dijkman A, Huisman C, Smit M, *et al.* Cardiac arrest in pregnancy: increasing use of perimortem caesarean section due to emergency skills training? *BJOG* 2010;**117**:282–7.

Goodwin A, Pearce A. The human wedge. A manoeuvre to relieve aortocaval compression during resuscitation in late pregnancy. *Anaesthesia* 1992;**47**:433–4.

Hayes I, Rathore R, Enohumah K, *et al.* Prevalence of factors associated with difficult intubation in early and late pregnancy: a prospective observational study. *Anaesthesia* 2011;**66**:234–5.

Izci B, Vennelle M, Liston W, *et al.* Sleep-disordered breathing and upper airway size in pregnancy and post-partum. *Eur Respir J* 2006;**27**:321–7.

Jeejeebhoy FM, Zelop CM, Windrim R, *et al.* Management of cardiac arrest in pregnancy: A systematic review. *Resuscitation* 2011;**82**(7):801–9.

Katz V, Balderston K, DeFreest M. Perimortem cesarean delivery: Were our assumptions correct? *Am J Obstet Gynecol* 2005;**192**:1916–21.

King S, Gabbott D. Maternal cardiac arrest – rarely occurs, rarely researched. *Resuscitation* 2011;**82**(7):795–6.

Nanson J, Elcock D, Williams M, Deakin C. Do physiological changes in pregnancy change defibrillation energy requirements? *Br J Anaesth* 2001;**87**:237–9.

Rees G, Willis B. Resuscitation in late pregnancy. *Anaesthesia* 1988;**43**:347–9.

Royal College of Obstetricians and Gynaecologists. Green Top Guideline No 56. Maternal Collapse in pregnancy and the puerpurium. January 2011.

NHS Quality Improvement Scotland. Scottish Confidential Audit of Severe Maternal Morbidity 5th Annual Report. Edinburgh, NHS Quality Improvement Scotland, 2007. http://www.nhshealthquality.org/nhsqis/files/SCASMM_ANNREP2007_MAY09.pdt.

Providing equity of critical and maternity care for the critically ill pregnant or recently pregnant woman. http://www.rcog.org.uk/files/rcog-corp/Prov_Eq_MatandCritCare.pdf.

Vanden Hoek TL, Morrison LJ, Shuster M, *et al.* Part 12 cardiac arrest in special situations: 2010 American Heart Association Guidelines for Cardiopulmonary Resuscitation and Emergency Cardiovascular Care. *Circulation* 2010;**122**:S829–S861.

CHAPTER 16

Drowning

Anthony J. Handley

Colchester Hospital University NHS Foundation Trust, Colchester, UK

OVERVIEW

- Drowning is a common cause of accidental injury and death, particularly in the young
- If attempting an aquatic rescue take care not to place yourself at risk of getting into difficulty and drowning
- Death due to drowning arises primarily as a consequence of hypoxia
- Initial treatments should prioritise airway and breathing interventions

---

Introduction

Worldwide, there are approximately 450,000 deaths each year from drowning. Most occur in low- and middle-income countries, but in 2006 there were 312 accidental deaths from drowning in the UK and 3582 in the USA, an annual incidence of 0.56 and 1.2 per 100,000 population respectively. Drowning is the leading cause of accidental death in Europe in young males. It occurs most commonly during the warmer summer months (Figure 16.1). Contrary to popular perception, nearly half of drowning cases occur in inland waterways. Drowning in a swimming pool is relatively rare (Figure 16.2).

Definition

Many definitions and sub-definitions of drowning exist which have resulted in confusion and inability to compare studies on management and outcome. To try and simplify matters, an advisory statement from the International Liaison Committee on Resuscitation (ILCOR) was published in 2003 under the title *Recommended Guidelines for Uniform Reporting of Data From Drowning. The "Utstein Style"*. In it, drowning was defined as a process rather than an event:

Drowning is a process resulting in primary respiratory impairment from submersion/immersion in a liquid medium. Implicit in this definition is that a liquid/air interface is present at the entrance of

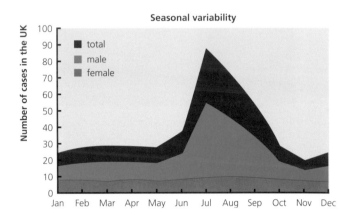

Figure 16.1 Seasonal variability for drowning.

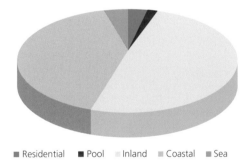

Figure 16.2 Location of drowning events.

the victim's airway, preventing the victim from breathing air. The victim may live or die after this process, but whatever the outcome, he or she has been involved in a drowning incident.

ILCOR also recommended that certain, ill-defined terms should be abandoned, including: wet/dry drowning; active/passive/silent drowning; secondary drowning; near-drowned; drowned.

The sequence of events in drowning that lead to death are summarised in Box 16.1.

The need for oxygen

When cardiac arrest occurs due to a primary cardiac cause (sudden cardiac death – SCD) the problem is one of failure to circulate blood that, at least initially, is well oxygenated. When cardiac arrest

ABC of Resuscitation, Sixth Edition. Edited by Jasmeet Soar, Gavin D. Perkins and Jerry Nolan.
© 2013 John Wiley & Sons, Ltd. Published 2013 by John Wiley & Sons, Ltd.

Box 16.1 **Sequence of events that occur following submersion**

The earlier that rescue occurs in this sequence the greater chance of survival

- Breath holding
- Laryngospasm
- Hypoxia and hypercarbia
- Swallowing
- Water inhalation
- Surfactant wash out, pulmonary hypertension, shunting
- Worsening hypoxia
- Loss of consciousness
- Death

occurs following drowning, the primary cause is hypoxia. In SCD, the priority of treatment is chest compression; in drowning, it is ventilation. Because around 70% of out-of-hospital cardiac arrests in developed countries are due to SCD, standard BLS guidelines are aimed at the majority case with the emphasis on chest compression. One of the important differences to be remembered when managing a case of drowning is that restoration of adequate ventilation is a prime objective.

The drowning victim

In many cases the victim has first to be rescued to dry land before definitive treatment can start. This presents dangers for the rescuer. Never enter the water unless absolutely necessary (Figure 16.3): consider reaching to the victim with a stick or throwing a rope or floating aid if the victim is near to land. If these will not reach and no boat is available, carefully weigh up the potential dangers of entering the water. If you have one, wear a lifejacket and take a floating aid with you. It is safer to go with another rescuer than on your own. Even then, be very wary of getting too close to a panicking victim who may grasp and pull you under the water. Even an apparently unconscious victim may 'recover' and grab you; the result can be two drowned victims rather than one.

Basic life support

Rescue breathing is possible in the water, but do not attempt this unless you have been trained in the technique. Mouth-to-nose ventilation may be used if it is difficult for the rescuer to pinch the victim's nose closed, support the head and open the airway in the water. Chest compression is not feasible.

Once on dry land, confirm cardiac arrest (unresponsive and not breathing normally), and position the victim supine with the head at the same level as the body (parallel with the shore). Laypersons trained in CPR should follow the standard CPR sequence and use the usual 30:2 compression:ventilation ratio. Healthcare providers, and those with a duty of care to drowning victims (such as lifeguards), should give 5 initial rescue breaths before continuing with a 30:2 compression:ventilation ratio.

Attempts at ventilation may be difficult due to increased resistance caused by water in the airways and pulmonary oedema. Chest

Safety	Consider your own safety first. Avoid entering the water	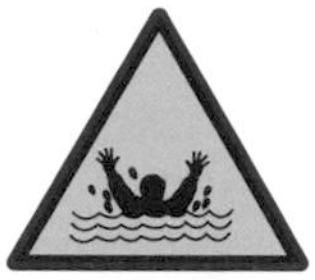
Talk	Talk to the victim, encourage them to help themselves	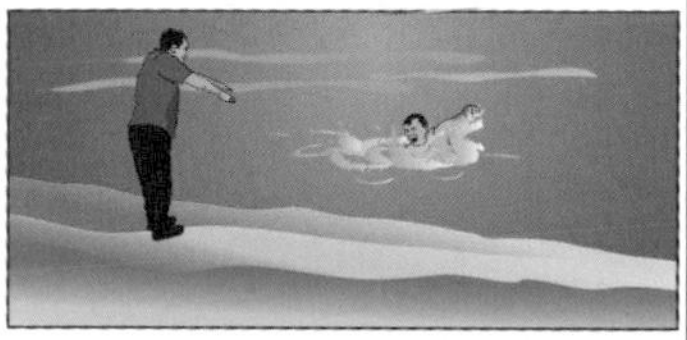
Reach	Reach with a stick or item of clothing	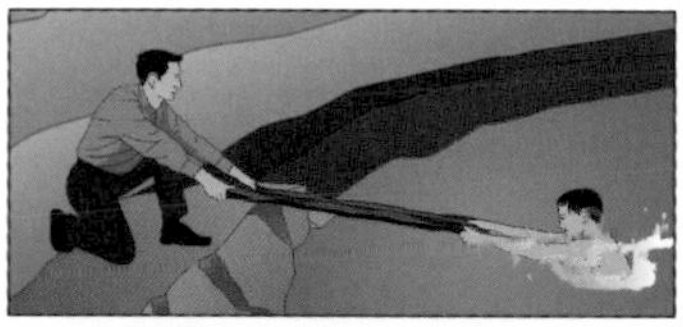
Throw	Throw a buoyant rescue aid (e.g. life ring or a ball) or a rope	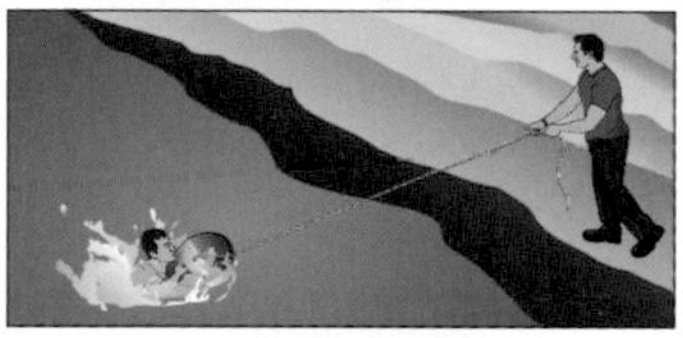
Boat	Consider if you could use a boat to assist the rescue	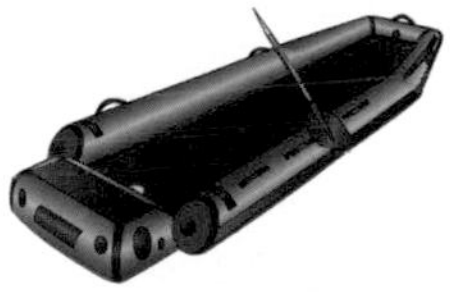
Swim with aid	Swim with an aid such as a life ring, torpedo buoy	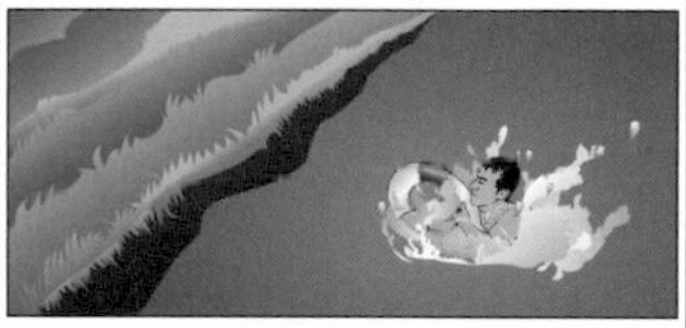
Swim and tow	Swim and tow the victim to shore	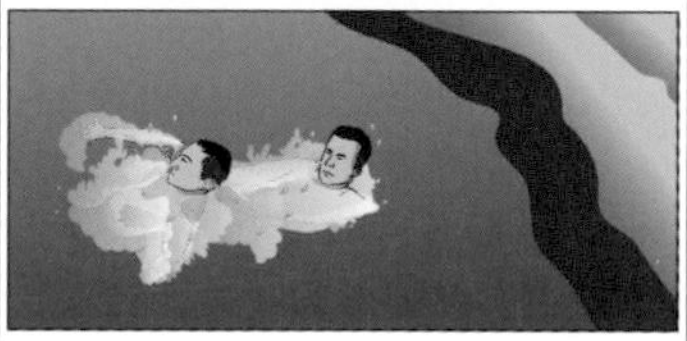

Figure 16.3 Rescue techniques.

compression may be hindered by reduced chest wall compliance, aggravated by hypothermia. These adverse conditions may be overcome by slowing down the rate of inflation and compression, but only as much as is necessary to achieve the necessary inflation and chest compression.

If oxygen is available this should be administered, provided it does not impede rescue breathing, for example by attaching to a resuscitation face mask.

Regurgitation of stomach contents is very common during resuscitation after drowning. If it occurs, the victim should be rolled onto the side, away from the rescuer, and the material cleared from the mouth.

Abdominal thrusts (Heimlich Manoeuvre) should only be used if there is clear evidence of solid material obstructing the airway. Never use as a routine procedure in drowning as this will only increase the chance of further gastric regurgitation and inhalation of fluid into the lungs. Chest compressions alone are often effective in clearing an airway obstruction.

Cervical spine injury

Contrary to popular belief, the incidence of cervical spine injury in drowning victims is surprisingly low (0.009%) unless there is a clear associated factor such as diving, water-slide use, signs of trauma or signs of alcohol intoxication. Although it is wise to keep the victim's head and torso in alignment during handling, unnecessary cervical spine immobilisation can interfere with opening the airway and may delay rescue breaths and the start of CPR. Routine stabilisation of the cervical spine in the absence of circumstances that suggest a spinal injury is not recommended.

Defibrillation

The first recorded ECG rhythm following cardiac arrest from drowning is less likely to be ventricular fibrillation (VF) than after SCD, but drowning may occur secondary to another cause of cardiac arrest, such as myocardial infarction or stroke. It can also occur, rarely but dramatically, particularly in young swimmers, as sudden collapse in the water. Some such cases are due to congenital, structural abnormalities (e.g. hypertrophic cardiomyopathy, arrhythmogenic right ventricular cardiomyopathy) or an ion channelopathy (e.g. long QT syndrome (LQTS); Brugada syndrome; catecholamine polymorphic ventricular tachycardia). In all these cases, VF may well be the presenting arrest rhythm and an automated external defibrillator (AED) should be sought as soon as possible whilst continuing uninterrupted CPR.

The victim should be removed from the water and the chest quickly dried to allow the AED electrode pads to adhere. The presence of some water on or around the victim does not pose an additional risk to the rescuer, but normal safety precautions should be observed.

Advanced life support

As soon as equipment, and those with the skills to use it, arrives:

1 Secure the airway by tracheal intubation, taking care to ensure optimal pre-oxygenation before intubation. Rapid-sequence induction with cricoid pressure will reduce the risk of aspiration.
2 Give oxygen in high concentration, preferably using positive end-expiratory pressure (PEEP).
3 Be particularly careful to differentiate the gasping, initial respiratory efforts of a victim recovering from drowning from the agonal gasps of one still in cardiac arrest: do not stop chest compression too soon (Box 16.2).
4 Institute all normal management for a victim of cardiac arrest.

> **Box 16.2 Don't confuse agonal breathing as a sign of life**
>
> A young, strong swimmer sustained a cardiac arrest in a swimming pool. During CPR slow deep and irregular breaths were noted, CPR was stopped and the victim died. The description is the characteristic appearance of agonal breathing. Agonal breathing is a sign of cardiac arrest. Do not stop CPR unless normal breathing or consciousness is restored.

Hypothermia and drowning

Victims of drowning may become hypothermic if they are submersed in icy water ($<5\,°C$). This can provide some protection against the effects of hypoxia and probably accounts for reports of victims (usually children) being successfully resuscitated after, perhaps, an hour under water. Extracorporeal membrane oxygenation (ECMO) has been used successfully following refractory cardiac arrest secondary to drowning, particularly when the victim is very cold.

Since therapeutic hypothermia is recommended for unconscious victims resuscitated from pre-hospital cardiac arrest, should hypothermia be reversed in a victim resuscitated after drowning? There is no good evidence-based guidance, but the International Life Saving Federation takes the pragmatic approach that such victims should be re-warmed until they reach a core temperature of $32–34\,°C$ during post-resuscitation intensive care.

Stopping CPR

Drowning (with or without hypothermia) is one situation in which attempts at resuscitation should be prolonged, even if the outlook seems hopeless. Neurologically intact survival has been reported after prolonged submersion times. Ideally, efforts to revive a drowning victim should continue until a senior medical doctor makes the decision to stop (see Box 16.2). Otherwise, follow the guidance of the Resuscitation Council (UK) and continue CPR until:

- Qualified help arrives and takes over
- The victim starts to show signs of regaining consciousness, such as coughing, opening his or her eyes, speaking, or moving purposefully AND starts to breathe normally, OR
- You become exhausted

Key modifications of the standard CPR sequence for healthcare providers is shown in Box 16.3.

> **Box 16.3 Modifications of standard CPR sequence for healthcare providers**
>
> *Basic life support*:
> 1 Start by giving rescue breathing (5 breaths)
> 2 Follow this with alternating cycles of 30 compressions to 2 rescue breaths
> 3 Give supplemental oxygen if available

Advanced life support:
1 Intubate early if equipment and training permit
2 Give high inspired oxygen concentrations
3 Use PEEP if possible
4 Rewarm if hypothermia present

Further reading

BBC News. Agonal breathing causes young swimmer's death. http://news.bbc .co.uk/1/hi/england/leicestershire/8535486.stm

Bierens JJLM (ed.). *Handbook on Drowning*. Berlin, Springer, 2006.

Layon AJ, Modell JH. Drowning: Update 2009. *Anesthesiology* 2009; **110**(6):1390–401.

Quan D, Szpilman JG, Wigginton JH *et al*. Recommended Guidelines for Uniform Reporting of Data From Drowning: The "Utstein Style". *Circulation* 2003;**108**:2565–74.

Soar J, Perkins GD, Abbas G, *et al*. European Resuscitation Council Guidelines for Resuscitation 2010 Section 8. Cardiac arrest in special circumstances: Electrolyte abnormalities, poisoning, drowning, accidental hypothermia, hyperthermia, asthma, anaphylaxis, cardiac surgery, trauma, pregnancy, electrocution. *Resuscitation* 2010;**81**(10):1400–33.

Szpilman D, Bierens J, Handley AJ, Orlowski JP. Current Concepts: Drowning. *N Engl J Med* 2012;**366**:2102–10.

CHAPTER 17

Trauma

Kate Crewdson[1] and David J. Lockey[1,2]

[1]North Bristol NHS Trust, Bristol, UK
[2]University of Bristol, Bristol, UK

OVERVIEW

- Major trauma is a significant cause of death and disability in the first four decades of life
- A standardised ABCDE approach underlies the principles of management of trauma patients
- Appropriate airway management is the priority for all trauma patients; failure to maintain an adequate airway remains a significant cause of preventable death in this patient group
- Provision of routine cervical spine immobilisation for all trauma patients is currently being questioned
- Novel therapies for the control of major haemorrhage and coagulopathy include haemostatic agents, early use of blood and blood products, and tranexamic acid
- Whilst traumatic cardiac arrest is universally associated with poor outcome, potential survivors may be identified from specific patient groups

Introduction

Major trauma is the term used to describe serious or multiple injuries associated with a significant possibility of death or disability. The term can be further subdivided into blunt or penetrating trauma. Blunt trauma describes injuries sustained from blunt force such as a road traffic collision or fall from height; penetrating trauma describes the injuries resulting from an object penetrating the body, commonly a knife or bullet. There are approximately 20,000 cases of major trauma in England each year, resulting in around 5400 deaths and many cases of permanent disability. The distribution and pattern of injury varies between countries, regions and over time. In the UK there has been a steady decrease in road traffic fatalities but an increase in penetrating trauma.

The resuscitation of trauma patients has, for many years, been heavily influenced by the ABCDE (Airway, Breathing, Circulation, Disability, Exposure) approach derived mainly from the American College of Surgeons' Advanced Trauma Life Support course. The

ABC of Resuscitation, Sixth Edition. Edited by Jasmeet Soar, Gavin D. Perkins and Jerry Nolan.
© 2013 John Wiley & Sons, Ltd. Published 2013 by John Wiley & Sons, Ltd.

course is taught in many countries to postgraduate physicians and other medical personnel but the main principles are embedded in standard undergraduate curricula. The approach taken is that in the initial management of trauma victims, the most lethal clinical problems are dealt with first. Thus, airway obstruction is dealt with before breathing problems, and breathing problems are dealt with before circulatory problems. This philosophy has been extrapolated in recent years to military practice where it was recognised that catastrophic haemorrhage from blast injuries may be more rapidly fatal than airway obstruction which has led to the term (C)ABC. This is rarely relevant to civilian practice. Priorities of care are the same wherever the patient is attended, that is in the pre-hospital environment, the district hospital or the trauma centre. Where the life-threatening problem cannot be immediately treated the patient needs to be rapidly transferred to a site where the problem can be addressed or a more advanced resource needs to be made available to attend the patient.

The concept of major trauma centres, which treat a large number of patients with the most severe injuries, is well established in the USA and some European countries including the UK. There is some evidence that centralisation of trauma care decreases mortality. Numerous reports have emphasised suboptimal trauma management in the UK and have provided the drive to develop trauma networks and trauma centres. Pre-hospital medical services are being developed throughout the UK, with the aim of providing interventions dictated by the immediate needs of patients without unnecessarily delaying their transfer to hospital.

Trauma patients require rapid assessment, triage and where appropriate, instigation of potentially life-saving interventions. The ABCDE approach to patient care provides a standardised framework that identifies the immediate needs of the patient whilst reducing potential for human error in a stressful situation by providing a basic structure for the personnel involved.

Airway management

Current practice

Prompt and effective airway assessment and management is essential for all trauma patients. Failure to maintain or secure an adequate airway and provide oxygenation in a timely fashion is a major cause of preventable death following significant injury (Box 17.1).

Simple airway manoeuvres such as a head-tilt and chin-lift, or a jaw thrust if cervical spine injury is anticipated, are used to open the patient's airway. If the patient is breathing, apply oxygen to the open airway and continue the primary survey. If the patient is not breathing or seems to have an obstructed airway, the airway remains the focus of the assessment until it is secured. Airway adjuncts such as an oropharyngeal or nasopharyngeal airway can help to restore airway patency. Do not use an oropharyngeal airway in a conscious patient as it will not be tolerated and is likely to stimulate vomiting and possible aspiration. Nasopharyngeal airways are better tolerated but insertion can be uncomfortable.

Supraglottic airway devices (SAD) are increasingly used by pre-hospital personnel. The main benefit of these devices is ease of insertion. They enable either spontaneous breathing or assisted ventilation. Recommendations from the UK Joint Royal Colleges Ambulance Liaison Committee (JRCALC) are that paramedics are trained to insert SADs instead of tracheal intubation. However, tracheal intubation with a cuffed tube remains the standard of airway care for those highly skilled in the technique. The positioning of a cuffed tube below the vocal cords will reduce the risk of airway soiling with blood or vomit. Injuries sustained to the head and neck may make intubation more difficult because of anatomical distortion, bleeding and airway oedema. Several emergency airway algorithms exist to improve the chances of successful intubation.

Further considerations

Rapid sequence induction (RSI) is a technique used by doctors to facilitate tracheal intubation in an emergency. Only those who are trained and skilled in the technique should attempt it. Oxygen is applied to pre-oxygenate the patient and maximise time to desaturation of arterial blood once the patient has been anaesthetised. An intravenous anaesthetic and short-acting neuromuscular blocker are used to induce anaesthesia and optimise conditions for intubation. As the drugs are given, a trained assistant applies backwards upwards pressure to the cricoid cartilage in an attempt to occlude the oesophagus and prevent passage of gastric contents into the lungs. In a standard RSI, the patient's lungs are not ventilated whilst the drugs take effect (usually 60–90 seconds) to further reduce the risk of aspiration; however, in the presence of significant lung injury, gentle lung inflation with oxygen will reduce the risk of hypoxaemia occuring during the procedure. Intubation is performed when the patient is fully anaesthetised and muscle relaxation has been achieved. Cricoid pressure is removed once the tracheal tube cuff has been inflated, correct positioning of the tube has been confirmed and ventilation has been established.

It is possible to establish ventilation in a non-breathing patient by accessing the trachea through the procedure of cricothyroidotomy. This technique is considered by most to be a last resort and is the final step in 'Can't Intubate, Can't Ventilate' guidelines. The procedure is best performed using a surgical technique, where a small horizontal incision is made, and a cuffed tube passed into the trachea. Needle cricothyroidotomy, in which a cannula is inserted through the cricothyroid membrane, is less successful.

Cervical spine immobilisation

Prehospital manual in-line stabilisation (MILS) of the cervical spine has been performed for several decades on patients who have sustained trauma, despite limited evidence for the practice. Patients are immobilised using a three-point technique involving application of a semi-rigid collar, placement on a spinal board, and lateral stabilisation of the neck and head with head blocks or sand bags. Overall, 2–5% of major trauma patients have cervical spine injury; this figure increases to 10% in comatose patients. Approximately 14% of cervical spine injuries are unstable. Until recently, all trauma patients have been immobilised, whether or not they had signs or symptoms of cervical spine injury; the rationale being that the consequences of worsening the injury may be catastrophic. This approach has recently been challenged. The practice of immobilising all trauma patients is not without risk: aside from significant discomfort to conscious patients and the possibility of pressure sores, it can significantly slow extrication time. Cervical immobilisation is associated with raised intracranial pressure and reduced cerebral perfusion pressure secondary to increased jugular venous pressure from spinal collars, which can be harmful in head-injured patients. The maximum forces applied to the cervical spine are likely to occur at the time of injury, and unlikely to be reproduced by controlled handling of the patient. This is particularly relevant to fully conscious patients, where muscle spasm following injury will provide better immobilisation, with fewer adverse effects, than artificially imposed immobilisation. A study of nearly 9000 alert and stable trauma patients demonstrated an incidence of 'clinically important' cervical spine injury in 1.7%, with 0.1% going on to develop neurological deficit. Subsequent neurological deterioration following controlled handling of the patient is unlikely. Unconscious patients, or those with a reduced conscious level, should be immobilised during transfer to prevent sudden uncontrolled movements of the head and cervical spine. (Figure 17.1)

Breathing

Current practice

Breathing is evaluated once the airway has been secured. The work of breathing, respiratory rate, oxygen saturation of arterial blood, and evidence of chest injury should be assessed in the spontaneously breathing patient. If the patient is not breathing adequately, bag-mask ventilation is used to provide oxygenation and ventilation until they either recover, or an individual with the appropriate skills can intubate the patient's trachea. Bag-mask

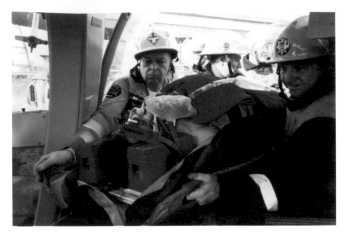

Figure 17.1 Cervical spine immobilisation: routine immobilisation for all trauma patients is now being questioned.

ventilation is a technique for providing positive pressure ventilation using a facemask, a self-inflating reservoir bag, and a low-pressure oxygen source. Sufficient time is left between ventilations to enable adequate exhalation and avoid hypercapnia.

Further considerations

The quality of ventilation provided is important, and adequate ventilation must occur to prevent hypoxia and hypercapnia. This is particularly important in head injured patients, where increased cerebral blood flow secondary to high carbon dioxide levels will increase intracranial pressure; hypoxia will also worsen the primary brain injury. Hyperventilation and consequent cerebral ischaemia must also be avoided. Failure of oxygenation and ventilation will result in respiratory demise and subsequent respiratory and cardiac arrest.

Circulation and haemorrhage control

Current practice

Assessment of the circulation includes measurement of the blood pressure, heart rate and capillary refill time. Cool peripheries and low urine output can also indicate inadequate perfusion pressure secondary to hypovolaemia or low cardiac output. Many patients, particularly the young, will maintain their systolic blood pressure (by vasoconstriction) despite losing up to 40% of their blood volume: hypotension is usually a late sign of hypovolaemia and a sign of decompensation. Significant hypovolaemia will precipitate shock – defined by tissue perfusion inadequate to meet the tissue's metabolic requirements; hypovolaemia is the most common form of shock occurring in trauma patients. Other forms of shock are neurogenic (e.g. spinal cord injury), cardiogenic, distributive (e.g. sepsis) and obstructive (e.g. pulmonary embolus).

Massive haemorrhage is a significant, and potentially preventable, cause of death in trauma patients. The immediate treatment is to stop any bleeding with an identifiable source, usually by the application of direct pressure, or occasionally with use of novel haemostatic agents. Fluid resuscitation in the management of trauma patients remains controversial; some guidelines recommend

using boluses of 250 ml of crystalloid fluid until a radial pulse can be palpated. In patients with head injury, the systolic blood pressure should be maintained between 90–100 mmHg.

Further considerations

Over recent years, most advances in the treatment of catastrophic bleeding have come from military experience involving the treatment of many patients with blast injuries. Attempts to control the major haemorrhage associated with many of these injuries has led to a shift in current practice, with the initial focus of resuscitation on controlling the bleeding. Use of tourniquets by the military has increased substantially and, anecdotally, this strategy has proven effective. (Figure 17.2)

The early use of blood and fresh frozen plasma as first line fluid therapy in hypovolaemic shock is becoming standard practice in many trauma centres and is replacing the practice of infusing large volumes of crystalloid, which is thought to worsen traumatic coagulopathy. The early use of tranexamic acid to reduce bleeding following major trauma follows a recent multicentre randomised controlled trial (Figure 17.3).

Disability

Current practice

Injury to the central nervous system is a major cause of death following trauma and all patients should undergo neurological assessment. Disability is assessed using either the Glasgow Coma Scale (GCS) (Table 17.1) or AVPU (**A**wake / responds to **P**ain / responds to **V**oice / **U**nresponsive) system.

Although GCS and AVPU are relatively blunt tools, they provide some indication of the patient's conscious level. If the patient has a GCS of 8 or less, it is generally considered that they will be unable to protect their own airway and require urgent airway management; a GCS of 8 correlates to V on the AVPU scale. In fact many patients with a GCS score greater than 8 are also at risk of airway compromise and serious intracerebral pathology. Much of the treatment of 'D' is managed by correct management of A, B and C. This provides

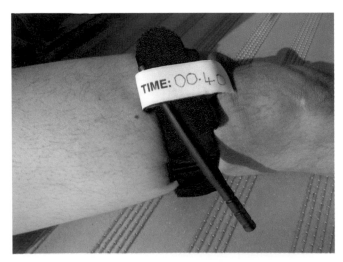

Figure 17.2 Combat Application Tourniquet (CAT): use of these devices remains controversial.

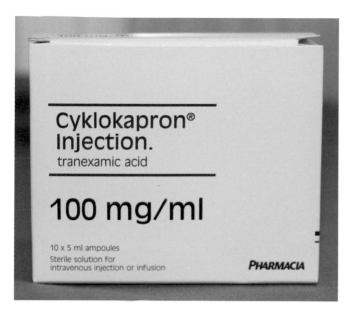

Figure 17.3 Tranexamic acid has been shown to reduce mortality in patients with acute traumatic coagulopathy.

Table 17.1 Glasgow Coma Scale.

	Response	Score
Best motor response	Obeys commands	6
	Localises pain	5
	Normal flexion withdrawal	4
	Abnormal flexion to pain	3
	Extension to pain	2
	No response	1
Best verbal response	Orientated	5
	Confused	4
	Inappropriate words	3
	Incomprehensible sounds	2
	No response	1
Best eye response	Eyes open	4
	Eyes open to speech	3
	Eyes open to pain	2
	No response	1

adequate neurological oxygenation, ventilation with normocarbia and perfusion. Persistently low or fluctuating GCS, seizures and recurrent vomiting are indications for further neurological assessment of the patient with computed tomography (CT).

Further considerations

Adequate oxygenation and avoidance of hypovolaemia and hypotension are important cerebral protection strategies. Other factors important in reducing the likelihood of secondary brain injury include positioning the patient 30° head up, securing the tracheal tube with tape, or ties passing above the ears, and removing the cervical collar to minimise venous congestion and subsequent raised intracranial pressure. Blood glucose is controlled tightly and hyperthermia avoided. Patients with significant head injury should be managed in specialist centres – the establishment of trauma networks should now ensure that this happens.

Traumatic cardiac arrest

Cardiac arrest in trauma has a high mortality but survival rates appear to be improving. The relative futility of attempting resuscitation in these patients is subject to continuing debate. Given that trauma occurs more commonly in the first four decades of life, the absence of underlying cardiac disease improves the chances of a better outcome if a potentially reversible cause of cardiac arrest is rapidly identified and treated. Those patients in whom hypoxaemia can be reversed, cardiac tamponade relieved or a tension pneumothorax decompressed, all in a timely fashion, have a reasonable chance of return of spontaneous circulation (ROSC). Immediate airway management and relief of hypoxia may result in ROSC in patients who have a respiratory arrest preceding the cardiac arrest. This pattern of events is likely in crush injury, hanging, drowning, electrocution and severe head or high spinal injury. Neurological outcome depends predominantly on the prevention of secondary brain injury; hypoxia and hypotension must be avoided. Hypovolaemic cardiac arrest is almost always fatal.

Further reading

American College of Surgeons. *Advanced Trauma Life Support Manual*, 8th edn. *ACS*, 2008.

Brohi K, Cole E, Hoffman K. Improving outcomes in the early phases after major trauma. *Curr Opin Crit Care* 2011;**17**:515–9.

CRASH-2 trial collaborators. Effects of tranexamic acid on death, vascular occlusive events, and blood transfusion in trauma patients with significant haemorrhage (CRASH-2): a randomised, placebo-controlled trial. *Lancet* 2010;**376**(9734):23–32.

Davenport R, Khan S. Management of major trauma haemorrhage: treatment priorities and controversies. *Br J Haematol* 2011;**155**:537–48.

National Confidential Enquiry into Patient Outcome and Death report. Trauma: Who Cares? 2007. http://www.ncepod.org.uk/2007t.htm.

Nolan JP (ed.) 2010 Resuscitation Guidelines. London, Resuscitation Council (UK), 2010.

Teasdale G, Jennett B. Assessment of coma and impaired consciousness. A practical scale. *Lancet* 1974;**2**(7872):81–4.

CHAPTER 18

Human Factors

Peter-Marc Fortune[1] and Andrew S. Lockey[2]

[1]Royal Manchester Children's Hospital, Manchester, UK
[2]Calderdale Royal Hospital, Halifax, UK

OVERVIEW

- Understand the importance of human factors in personal and team performance
- Have an overview understanding of how medical accidents occur
- Understand the limitations of communication and have some simple tools to improve personal communication
- Understand the concept of 'situation awareness' and its importance to good decision making

---

Introduction

In the year ending June 2009, there were just under one million incidents reported to the Department of Health by NHS facilities in England. Over 90% of these resulted in no harm or minimal harm to patients. However, on just under 70,000 occasions patients suffered significant harm; 7773 of these suffered permanent damage and 3735 people died.

Human factors (HF) are the environmental and behavioural elements that influence the way that people, or teams of people, interact with one another and the equipment and devices they use. In the analysis of healthcare critical incidents, they are found to play a causal role in 60–80% of cases. Extrapolating from the figures given here, these factors are likely to contribute to more than 2200 patient deaths each year.

Traditional resuscitation training used to focus on the factual knowledge and practical (technical) skills that are required to assess and treat the collapsed patient. There is now an increasing trend of instruction in HF within resuscitation courses and in general in the NHS as part of the patient safety agenda. It is against this background that this chapter has been included in this book.

A full discussion of HF is outside the scope of this book. The content is focused on three specific areas that are directly relevant to those attending and managing collapsed patients on an infrequent basis: how accidents occur, communication issues and the concept of situation awareness.

Nature of accidents

It is vital to recognise that we all make errors. Sometimes, even when multiple stops and checks have been put into place, things can still go wrong. On occasions, accidents may even occur as a consequence of the procedures put in place to prevent them.

The error chain

The key to recognising, understanding and preventing accidents is to understand that people do not seek to cause them. Bad or catastrophic events usually occur because a series of small errors or adverse circumstances that come together at a particular time and place. This creates a situation where the final error that triggers the accident is either inevitable or occurs through an action which seems entirely reasonable at the time. This concept, known as an error chain, was originally described by James Reason. It is also often referred to as 'the Swiss cheese model' and is shown in Figure 18.1.

Each layer of cheese represents a layer of defence such as a protocol, procedure or an environmental condition that serves to prevent an accident occurring. The holes represent the imperfections. When all the holes line up an accident occurs. Accidents can be prevented by identifying and plugging these holes. A clinical example of how this may be achieved is shown in Box 18.1.

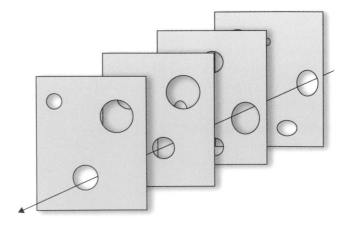

Figure 18.1 James Reason's Swiss cheese model of an error chain. (Reproduced from Reason J. Human error: models and management. BMJ. 2000 March 18; 320: 768–770, with permission from BMJ Publishing Group Ltd.)

ABC of Resuscitation, Sixth Edition. Edited by Jasmeet Soar, Gavin D. Perkins and Jerry Nolan.

Box 18.1 **Identifying and plugging 'holes'**

At one trust it was noted that a number of incidents had occurred secondary to problems with emergency airway equipment. On closer examination it was found that the handles and the blades of the laryngoscopes on the affected trolleys were made by different manufacturers and were incompatible. The hole in the 'physical' layer was closed by standardising the type of laryngoscope used across the trust.

Note that this safeguard may still be overridden by a member of staff ordering an incorrect replacement for a used handle or blade. Preventing such behaviours depends in part on adequate training. However, good application of HF principles would also consider strategies to address softer factors, for example incorrect replacement orders may be placed when people are tired, distracted or unfocused for some other reason.

Individual fitness to work is a critical issue and is often poorly considered because of a desire not to let colleagues down. This has been recognized by the airline industry who introduced a personal self-screening checklist (*IM SAFE*) to highlight when a person should consider that they may not fit for work. This list is detailed in Table 18.1.

In practice everyone needs to maintain vigilance for the presence of factors that might be seen as a hole in the cheese. They are often known as 'Red Flags' and they herald a weakening defence. When they are spotted it is vital they are shared with the team so that actions can be undertaken (or omitted) to prevent them becoming part of an error chain.

Communication

Issues around communication feature in almost every critical event. To understand why this occurs, it is useful to consider a simple model of communication like that shown in Table 18.2.

When we talk to one another we are trying to share or explore a concept or idea. On the part of the speaker (source) they have a model in their head of the issue being discussed and will base what they say on their view of that model (encoding). Their words pass from them, through a channel (room air or a telephone) to a listener (receiver) who will then interpret the words they hear and fit them into their own current model (decoding). Examples of how common situations can adversely affect this process are shown in Figure 18.2.

Notice that feedback is a very powerful tool that can be used at all times to check that a message has been received and understood.

Table 18.1 IM SAFE checklist for fitness to work.

|---|---|
Illness	Could my illness affect my performance at work?
Medication	Am I taking any medications that might affect my performance at work?
Stress	Am I stressed? Is it sufficient to draw me away from my focus at work?
Alcohol	Has the effects of last night worn off? Think before you drink! The night before an on-call is not the night to overindulge!
Fatigue	Have I had enough sleep recently?
Eating	Have I eaten appropriately to prepare me for a working day?

Table 18.2 Common situations and their effect on the communication process.

Situation (stage of communication)	Consequence	Potential solutions
Channel: A noisy environment	The listener does not hear the speaker clearly. Missing or corrupted information may be guessed either consciously or unconsciously consequently distorting the meaning the speaker meant to convey.	Move to a quieter environment Avoid irrelevant conversations Utilise feedback
Channel & Encode/Decode: Language barriers	One of the two speakers is not using their first language or messages are replayed through an interpreter	Use professional interpreters Utilise feedback
Encode/Decode: Mental Models Differ (see situation awareness below)	Meaning of spoken words are misinterpreted because the listener does not have the same information and experience as the speaker	Utilise Briefings Use structured communications Utilise feedback

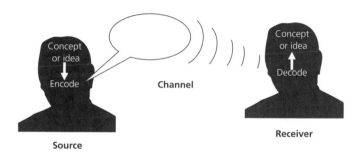

Figure 18.2 A simple model of speech communication.

It requires the listener to provide a confirmatory response to the speaker of what they have just heard (ideally in their own words). Thus when attending a patient collapse the lead person may say 'Can someone get help please!' A useful response from a nearby colleague would be 'No problem, I'll put out a cardiac arrest call and come back'.

At a patient collapse, those present expect the sequence of ABC to be followed. This serves two purposes: (1) it maintains the correct priorities and (2) it keeps the team members focused on the same principles. The use of structured communication offers the same advantages. The SBAR structure that is now used in many clinical communications is particularly helpful in the emergency situation as it guides appropriate prioritisation, focus and brevity. A summary of SBAR is shown in Table 18.3. Extensive supporting material may be found on the NHS Institute for Innovation and Improvement website.

Failure to escalate

A common theme in clinical incidents is also a failure to escalate to senior staff appropriately. This sometimes occurs because junior staff do not feel able to speak up. This may arise because of a fear of

Table 18.3 The SBAR communication tool.

Item	Definition	Example
Situation	A one sentence description of need	I'm ringing you about a collapsed patient
Background	Details that give information to make the assessment	I am the on-call medical doctor. I have been called to see a 71-year-old man in surgical outpatients. He has a known history of ischaemic heart disease. He is cold, clammy and breathless. I am giving him oxygen and moving him to the Emergency Department
Assessment	Your position on the issue	He needs to be reviewed by a senior doctor.
Recommendation	Your specific method for solving the problem	I would like you to attend urgently please

Table 18.4 The PACE acronym for escalating concern.

Stage	Level of concern
P – Probe	I think you need to know what is happening
A – Alert	I think something bad might happen
C – Challenge	I know something bad will happen
E – Emergency	I will not let it happen

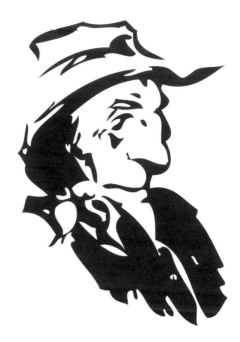

Figure 18.3 What do you see?

speaking out of turn or looking stupid. Poor leaders promote such behaviours by ignoring, snapping or ridiculing such feedback. None of these behaviours have any place in a safe environment and it is absolutely vital that anyone who feels they have an important piece of information that might prevent an accident feels able to share it.

In the aviation industry, crew are advised to use a structured approach to escalating a concern using the acronym PACE, shown in Table 18.4.

Consider the application of this structure where an observer at a resuscitation attempt notices that the oxygen piping has become disconnected from the wall outlet:

They begin by making a *Probing* statement 'Has anyone noticed that the oxygen is disconnected?'.

In the absence of a response this may become more directed by raising an *Alert*: 'Excuse me! The oxygen line is not connected to the supply properly.'

If this fails the person should move to a *Challenge*. Ideally this should involve the use of a key persons title or name: 'Doctor Smith, your oxygen line is not connected to the supply!'.

Finally if all else has failed and an *Emergency* is presenting, a physical intervention may be required: The observer might tap the resuscitators shoulder or wave a hand directly in their line of vision. They <u>must</u> grab their attention. 'You must connect the oxygen line now!'

Situation awareness

Situation awareness refers to the mental models that we have in our head of the world around us. We use it to plan our actions and we base our communications with others upon it (see above). It is not difficult to see that if this model is wrong then disaster may ensue.

Obtaining complete and accurate information can be very difficult. At the simplest level our eyes often deceive us. Is the illustration in Figure 18.3 a cowboy looking away or an old lady?

Good teams talk to one another; they don't just assume they are all following the same principles. Key issues must always be shared, ideally in a formal briefing.

In a resuscitation attempt, vocalising the algorithms as they are actioned is an excellent way of ensuring both concordance of thought and allowing for others to highlight oversights.

A marker that may indicate inadequate situation awareness is the acquisition of information that does not fit well into your current model. In many situations such information is disregarded or an unusual explanation is concocted to make it fit. This is known as confirmation bias. Don't fall into the trap! If new facts don't fit, go back to the beginning. Ask yourself, could the working diagnosis be wrong?

Summary

Most accidents happen secondary to a series of errors that come together to make an accident occur. People do not intend to do harm, and at the time they act inappropriately their actions will have seemed entirely reasonable to them (or they wouldn't have carried them out).

Patient harm can be reduced by ensuring accurate and timely communication. Further gains follow by ensuring that everyone continually re-examines the information they have and shares any concerns they have with the team. Feedback and structured communications are useful tools to achieve the these goals in the emergency situation.

Further reading

Civil Aviation Authority. Safety Sense Leaflet – Pilot Health, Number 24. Civil Aviation Authority, 2008.

Dekker S. *The Field Guide to Understanding Human Error*. Ashgate, 2008.

Flin R, O'Connor P, Crichton M. *Safety at the Sharp End – A Guide to Non-Technical Skills*. Ashgate, 2008.

National Patient Safety Agency (NPSA). National Reporting and Learning System Quarterly Data, Issue 14, November 2009.

NHS Institute for Innovation and Improvement. http://www.institute.nhs .uk/innovation/innovation/introduction.html.

Norris EM, Lockey AS. Human factors in resuscitation training. *Resuscitation* 2012;**83**(4):423–7.

Reason J. *Human error: models and management. BMJ* 2000;**320**:768–70.

CHAPTER 19

CPR Devices

Gavin D. Perkins[1] and Jerry Nolan[2]

[1]Warwick Medical School, University of Warwick, Coventry, UK
[2]Royal United Hospital, Bath, UK

OVERVIEW

- High quality, uninterrupted cardiopulmonary resuscitation (CPR) is critical to ensuring optimal outcomes from cardiac arrest
- CPR feedback and prompt devices can improve the quality of manual CPR
- Mechanical chest compression devices can deliver high-quality consistent CPR. Their effect on outcome is uncertain
- Active compression–decompression (ACD) CPR improves haemodynamics but not survival
- The combination of ACD–CPR and the impedance threshold device (ITD) may improve survival after out-of-hospital cardiac arrest

Box 19.1 **Characteristics of high-quality CPR**

- Compression depth 5–6 cm
- Compression rate 100–120 min^{-1}
- Minimise interruptions in compressions
- Ensure full chest re-coil between compressions
- Avoid hyperventilation

The importance of high-quality cardiopulmonary resuscitation

The performance of high-quality, uninterrupted chest compressions is an important determinant of outcome from cardiac arrest (Box 19.1). Observational studies have shown that chest compression depth influences shock success, return of spontaneous circulation rates (ROSC) and survival. Higher chest compression rates (up to 125 min^{-1}) are linked to improved ROSC. In animal models, failing to release pressure between compressions reduces coronary blood flow, which may have a negative effect on outcomes. Similarly, hyperventilation raises mean intrathoracic pressure, which reduces coronary perfusion and worsens outcome. CPR fraction (the proportion of resuscitation time spent performing chest compressions) is also a strong predictor of survival. Despite the prominence of CPR technique on outcome, observational studies provide consistent evidence of poor-quality CPR in clinical practice.

Cardiopulmonary resuscitation feedback and prompt devices

Cardiopulmonary resuscitation feedback and prompt devices aim to improve the performance of resuscitation skills by CPR providers (Table 19.1). Cardiopulmonary resuscitation feedback devices give information on the quality of CPR as it is performed, either through a visual display or audio instructions. Cardiopulmonary resuscitation prompt devices provide guidance to perform specific actions (e.g. sequence of CPR, audible beep for compression rate). The devices range in complexity from a simple metronome to an advanced defibrillator providing audio and visual feedback and prompts (Figure 19.1).

The more sophisticated devices assess CPR performance by measuring transthoracic impedance through defibrillation electrodes or through the use of an accelerometer (a small device placed on the sternum) or a combination of both. Measurement of transthoracic impedance enables chest compression rate, compression fraction and ventilation rate to be calculated. The addition of an accelerometer enables compression depth and completeness of release between compressions to be quantified (Figure 19.2).

A systematic review of the evidence for CPR feedback and prompt devices conducted as part of the International Liaison Committee for Resuscitation (ILCOR) review of resuscitation science in 2010, concluded that there is good evidence supporting the use of CPR feedback/prompt devices during CPR training to improve CPR skill acquisition and retention. Their use in clinical practice as part of an overall strategy may also be beneficial. The review highlights that accelerometers underestimate chest compression depth when CPR is performed on a soft surface such as a mattress as they do not differentiate between chest compression and mattress compression.

Since the publication of this review, a large cluster randomised study in the US examined the use of CPR feedback technology in out of hospital cardiac arrest. Although CPR feedback technology improved CPR quality, there was no difference in ROSC rates or survival to discharge. However, baseline CPR performance and survival was higher than that observed in many communities, thus leaving limited opportunity for CPR process improvement

ABC of Resuscitation, Sixth Edition. Edited by Jasmeet Soar, Gavin D. Perkins and Jerry Nolan.
© 2013 John Wiley & Sons, Ltd. Published 2013 by John Wiley & Sons, Ltd.

Table 19.1 Summary of different CPR feedback/prompt technology and their applications. Filled circle, currently available technology; empty circle, technology in early development phase.

CPR feedback/ prompt technology	Chest compressions				Ventilation		Patient	
	Depth	Rate	Recoil	Interruptions	Ventilation rate	Oesophageal intubation	Cardiac output	ROSC
Metronome		•						
Pressure sensor		•	•					
Impedance		•			•	○		○
Accelerometer	•	•	•					
Magnetic field	○	○	○	○				
End tidal CO_2					•	•	•	•
Rescuer movement detection	○	○	○	○				

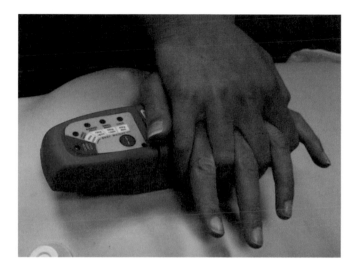

Figure 19.1 Simple CPR feedback/prompt device.

to affect outcome. The time taken for rhythm analysis with an automated external defibrillator may have negated the effect of CPR quality improvement. Finally, the study investigated a single CPR feedback system. Whether other systems or the addition of post-event debriefing of emergency medical services (EMS) staff would influence outcomes remains to be determined. Further trials of CPR feedback technology during in- and out-of-hospital cardiac arrest are in progress.

Mobile phones

The now almost universal carriage of mobile smart phones positions them as a potentially useful adjunct for CPR practice. Applications that support initial training, feedback/prompts during resuscitation and audit of outcomes have been developed (Table 19.2 and Figure 19.3).

Mechanical chest compression devices

Mechanical chest compression devices automate the process of chest compression. Advantages of mechanical CPR devices are the provision of consistent quality, non-fatiguing chest compressions and freeing up a member of the resuscitation team (Box 19.2). Potential disadvantages are interruption during CPR to deploy the device, which may increase no flow time (the time without

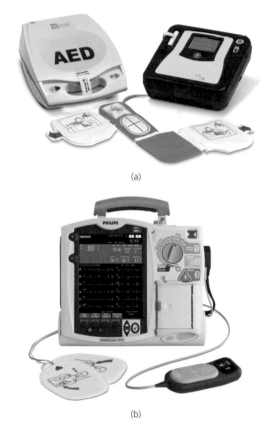

(a)

(b)

Figure 19.2 Sophisticated CPR feedback/prompt devices integrated with defibrillators. Reproduced by permission of ZOLL Medical Corporation. Reproduced by permission of Philips Electronics UK Limited.

chest compressions) and the potential for chest/visceral injuries; however, these need to be considered in the context of overall survival. Two main devices are in use clinically: the AutoPulse and the LUCAS device.

Box 19.2 **Potential advantages and disadvantages of mechanical CPR**

- Potential advantages
  - Consistent quality of CPR
  - CPR quality does not fatigue

- Releases a member of the resuscitation team from manual compressions
- Shock delivery during chest compression
- Can be deployed in confined spaces
• Potential disadvantages
  - Interruptions to CPR during deployment
  - Risk of chest wall and visceral injuries

AutoPulse

The AutoPulse device consists of a load distributing band (LDB) that is placed around the chest and backboard. The LDB tightens around the chest and then loosens to allow passive decompression; this cycle occurs at 80 per minute. The device adjusts the LDB to the size of the patient and distributes the compressive load over the anterior chest (Figure 19.4). Animal and human studies show improved physiological parameters compared with manual CPR.

The AutoPulse has been examined in two large-scale randomised controlled trials. The ASPIRE trial showed worse neurological outcomes and a trend toward worse survival in the AutoPulse arm compared to the manual CPR group. The follow-up trial (CIRC trial) compared AutoPulse with manual CPR in CPR-optimised EMS systems. Early results indicate treatment with Autopulse led to similar outcomes to the manual CPR group.

LUCAS

LUCAS provides both chest compression and active decompression. It consists of a silicon rubber suction cup that is applied to the chest

and an electric motor mounted on two legs which are connected to a stiff back plate (Figure 19.5). The original LUCAS device was gas driven (oxygen/air) but has been superseded by a battery driven device (LUCAS-2). This development has overcome the logistical requirement to carry compressed gas to power the device and initial concerns about the development of high oxygen concentrations in confined spaces. The device compresses the chest between 4 and 5 cm at a rate of 100 compressions per minute with an equal amount of time being spent in compression and decompression. Animal and human studies have shown improved physiological parameters compared with manual CPR. Studies focusing on clinical outcomes have produced mixed/inconclusive results. The results of two large-scale randomised controlled trials are awaited.

Current status

At present there is insufficient evidence to recommend the routine use of mechanical chest compression devices. Situations where deployment may be considered include where it is physically difficult to perform CPR e.g. cardiac catheter lab, confined spaces, during prolonged resuscitation attempts or to maintain circulation after cardiac death as a bridge to organ retrieval. There is an urgent need for definitive clinical and cost effectiveness trials to confirm or refute the routine use of mechanical chest-compression devices during resuscitation.

Active compression–decompression CPR

Active compression–decompression CPR (ACD–CPR) is achieved with a hand-held device that incorporates a suction cup that enables the chest to be lifted actively during decompression (Figure 19.6).

Table 19.2 Mobile phone technology can support each link of the chain of survival.

Early access	Early CPR	Early defibrillation	Post-resuscitation care and audit
Call EMS	Adjunct to dispatcher CPR	Locate nearest AED	Checklists
Mobile phone tracking to locate patient	CPR feedback/prompt instructions	Dispatch community AED response	Audit: transmit CPR quality data for review
Mobile phone tracking to detect nearest response		Monitor ECG	Audit: collate and submit code summaries
SMS to activate community responders			

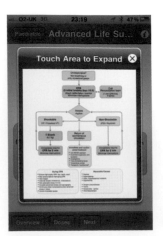

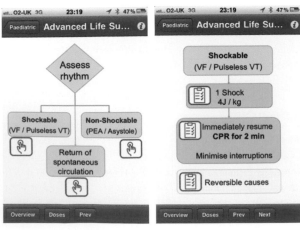

Figure 19.3 The i-resus application contains the Resuscitation Council (UK) CPR guidelines in an easy to navigate format. Reproduced with the kind permission of the Resuscitation Council (UK).

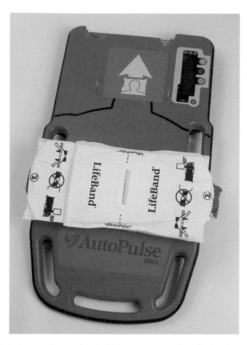

Figure 19.4 Autopulse mechanical chest compression device. Reproduced by permission of ZOLL Medical Corporation.

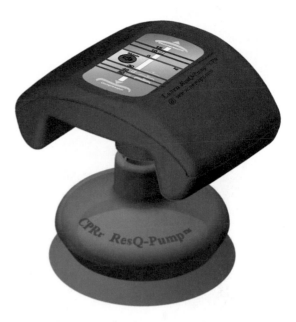

Figure 19.6 Active compression–decompression device. Reproduced with permission from Advanced Circulatory Systems Inc.

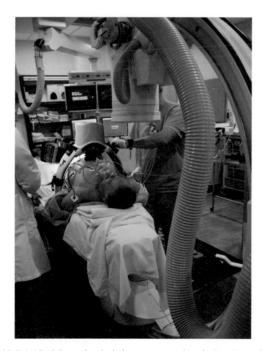

Figure 19.5 LUCAS-2 mechanical chest compression device. Reproduced by permission of Physio-Control, Inc.

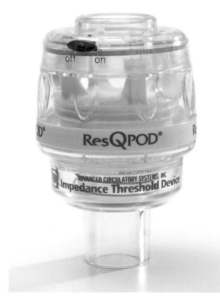

Figure 19.7 Impedance threshold device. Reproduced with permission from Advanced Circulatory Systems Inc.

The active decompression reduces intrathoracic pressure, which increases venous return to the heart, increases cardiac output and increases coronary and cerebral perfusion pressures during the compression phase. In some clinical studies ACD–CPR improved haemodynamics compared with standard CPR. In three randomised studies, ACD–CPR improved long-term survival after out-of-hospital cardiac arrest; however, in five other randomised studies, ACD–CPR made no difference to outcome. A meta-analysis of 10 trials of out-of-hospital cardiac arrest and two of in-hospital cardiac arrest showed no survival benefit for ACD–CPR compared with standard CPR. The efficacy of ACD–CPR may be highly dependent on the quality and duration of training. In comparison with standard CPR, ACD–CPR is more tiring for the rescuer. ACD–CPR causes more rib and sternal fractures than standard CPR. Although only a few enthusiasts use manual ACD–CPR, the ACD principle is incorporated in LUCAS, which is in more common use.

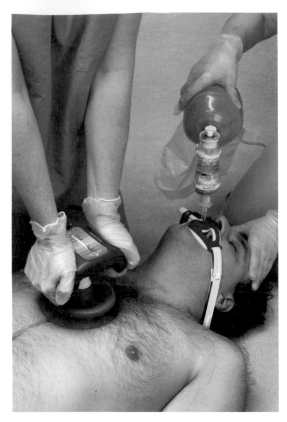

Figure 19.8 Combined use of active compression–decompression device and impedance threshold device. Reproduced with permission from Advanced Circulatory Systems Inc.

Impedance threshold device

The impedance threshold device (ITD) is a valve that limits air entry into the lungs during chest recoil between chest compressions (Figure 19.7). This decreases intrathoracic pressure and increases venous return to the heart. When used with a tracheal tube and ACD–CPR, the ITD acts synergistically to enhance venous return during active decompression. The ITD has also been used during conventional CPR with a tracheal tube, supraglottic airway device or facemask. Most animal studies have shown improved haemodynamics during CPR when using the ITD. One recent randomised trial showed that the use of an ITD in combination with ACD–CPR improved survival to hospital discharge and at 1 year in adult OHCA patients. In contrast, a randomised trial comparing an active ITD with a sham ITD in OHCA patients treated with standard CPR documented no difference in survival with good neurological function. The discrepancy in the results in the studies might be explained by the unblinded nature of the ACD–CPR study or may simply reflect that the ITD is effective only when combined with ACD–CPR (Figure 19.8). Based on these conflicting results, the ITD has not been implemented widely.

Further reading

Aufderheide TP, Frascone RJ, Wayne MA, *et al.* Standard cardiopulmonary resuscitation versus active compression-decompression cardiopulmonary resuscitation with augmentation of negative intrathoracic pressure for out-of-hospital cardiac arrest: a randomised trial. *Lancet* 2011;**377**:301–11.

Aufderheide TP, Nichol G, Rea TD, *et al.* A trial of an impedance threshold device in out-of-hospital cardiac arrest. *N Engl J Med* 2011;**365**:798–806.

Deakin CD, Nolan JP, Soar J, *et al.* European Resuscitation Council Guidelines for Resuscitation 2010 Section 4. Adult advanced life support. *Resuscitation* 2010;**81**:1305–52.

Lim SH, Shuster M, Deakin CD, *et al.* Part 7: CPR techniques and devices: 2010 International Consensus on Cardiopulmonary Resuscitation and Emergency Cardiovascular Care Science with Treatment Recommendations. *Resuscitation* 2010;**81**(Suppl 1):e86–92.

Perkins GD, Brace S, Gates S. Mechanical chest-compression devices: current and future roles. *Curr Opin Crit Care* 2010;**16**:203–210.

Yeung J, Meeks R, Edelson D, *et al.* The use of CPR feedback/prompt devices during training and CPR performance: A systematic review. *Resuscitation* 2009;**80**:743–751.

CHAPTER 20

Resuscitation in Sport

Carl Gwinnutt

Salford Royal Hospital NHS Foundation Trust, Salford, UK

OVERVIEW

- Underlying cardiovascular disease is the main cause of SCD in athletes
- A ventricular arrhythmia is usually the cause of cardiac arrest
- Early recognition and use of a defibrillator increases the chances of successful resuscitation
- Cardiac arrest in sport secondary to trauma has a poor outcome
- Identification of and treatment of a reversible cause is the key to resuscitation

---

Resuscitation in sport

Cardiac arrest occurring during sporting activity is fortunately relatively rare. Most cases are non-traumatic (80%) and occur in young males. Of these non-traumatic causes, 90% are cardiac in origin (Table 20.1). Over the past 30 years the incidence of cardiac arrest during sporting activity has increased, with cardiovascular disease being the main aetiology. The term sudden cardiac death (SCD) is used to describe such an event and is defined as 'natural death due to cardiac causes, heralded by abrupt loss of consciousness within one hour of the onset of acute symptoms; pre-existing heart disease may have been known to have been present but the time and mode of death are unexpected' (European Society of Cardiology). In athletes this can occur both during competition and training and the incidence varies: in high school and college athletes, studies from the USA report 0.5 cases per 100,000 athletes, where as in some areas of Italy, the incidence is as high as 3.6 cases per 100,000. Under the age of 35 years, the aetiology is predominantly congenital or inherited abnormalities, whereas over the age of 35 years, the vast majority are caused by coronary artery disease. Within this latter group, there is a 10-fold increase in incidence amongst those who engage in infrequent vigorous exercise, with 1:1500 'joggers' sustaining sudden cardiac death compared with 1:50,000 marathon runners, and males are ten times more likely to be affected than females. The more common cardiac causes of cardiac arrest are covered below (see also Table 2.1 in Chapter 2).

ABC of Resuscitation, Sixth Edition. Edited by Jasmeet Soar, Gavin D. Perkins and Jerry Nolan.
© 2013 John Wiley & Sons, Ltd. Published 2013 by John Wiley & Sons, Ltd.

Non-traumatic cardiac arrest

Hypertrophic cardiomyopathy (HCM)

In most parts of the world, HCM is the commonest cause of SCD during sport, the exception being Italy (see below). It is an inherited cardiac abnormality, autosomal dominant with variable expression, affecting around 0.2% of the population resulting in hypertrophy of the interventricular septum and anterior wall of the left ventricle. At a cellular level, there is hypertrophy of individual myocytes and myocardial fibre disarray, the degree of which predisposes to electrical re-entry and sudden death. Unfortunately, the first evidence of HCM in an athlete is often at autopsy, after a cardiac arrest during exercise, due to a ventricular arrhythmia. Occasionally, syncope may occur after exercise as a result of a ventricular tachyarrhythmia, left ventricular outflow obstruction reducing cardiac output, a paradoxical fall in blood pressure or a vasovagal attack. A routine 12-lead ECG will show abnormalities in more than 90% patients; these may include left axis deviation, abnormal T-wave inversion, pathological Q waves, and increased R- or S-wave amplitude in the anterior chest leads (Figure 20.1).

It is important that this condition is not confused with 'athlete's heart' where significant changes are induced as a result of extreme training. The European Society of Cardiology recognises the following as training-related ECG changes: sinus bradycardia, first degree heart block, incomplete right bundle branch block, early repolarisation and isolated left ventricular hypertrophy (LVH) by voltage criteria. Other changes favouring the diagnosis of athlete's heart include a reduction in LV mass after a short period of deconditioning, a LV end-diastolic diameter greater than 55 mm (compared with less than 45 mm in HCM) and normal Doppler-derived indices of LV diastolic filling and relaxation. Cardiac MR imaging may be of value in the diagnosis of HCM by detecting segmental LV hypertrophy and delayed gadolinium enhancement, due to fibrotic replacement of myocytes, and also in those patients in whom poor echo images are obtained.

Congenital coronary artery anomalies (CCAA)

This is the second commonest cause of SCD in athletes, usually due to the left main coronary artery arising from the right sinus of Valsalva. One theory is that because the artery passes between the aorta and the pulmonary trunk, it is compressed as the aorta expands during exercise. Victims may present with exercise-induced

Table 20.1 Aetiology of cardiac arrest in athletes.

Non-traumatic (80%)

Cardiac (90%)	Hypertrophic cardiomyopathy
	Congenital coronary artery anomalies
	Arrhythmogenic right ventricular cardiomyopathy (AVRC)
	Ischaemic heart disease
	Ion channel disorders
Non-cardiac (10%)	Heat stroke
	Asthma
	Illicit drugs
	Intracranial haemorrhage

Traumatic (20%)

Neurological	Head or cervical spine injury
Cardiovascular	Haemorrhage
	Commotio cordis
Respiratory	Tension pneumothorax
	Pulmonary contusion
Others	Lightning strike
	Drowning
	Suicide

ischaemia (chest pain) and syncope (arrhythmias); however, their resting ECG may be normal.

Arrhythmogenic right ventricular cardiomyopathy (ARVC)

This is an inherited disorder, autosomal dominant, and 30–50% of victims have a family history. It seems to be particularly prevalent in Italy, most probably as a result of a pre-participation screening programme whereby athletes with HCM have been identified and prevented from participation in sport, thereby changing the apparent aetiology of SCD. AVRC causes progressive atrophy of the myocytes with fibro-fatty replacement, usually within the free wall of the right ventricle. The commonest initial presentation is syncope with ventricular tachycardia (VT). There are various associated ECG abnormalities: T-wave inversion in leads V1–3, right bundle branch block, presence of an epsilon wave (a notched deflection after the QRS complex) (Figure 20.2), and frequent premature ventricular contractions on a 24-h ECG recording.

Coronary artery disease (CAD)

In those over the age of 35 years, CAD accounts for 80% of cases of SCD. It occurs mainly in males, participating in individual sports, usually running. They often have pre-existing identified risk factors: hypertension, hypercholesterolaemia, diabetes and smoking. Around 50% have experienced previous cardiac symptoms such as angina. At post mortem, all have significant disease of one or more main coronary arteries.

Ion channel disorders (channelopathies)

About 20% of cases of SCD will have an apparently structurally normal heart at post-mortem examination. A proportion of these victims will have an underlying ion channel disorder such as long QT syndromes (LQTS), Brugada syndrome, catecholaminergic polymorphic ventricular tachycardia (CPVT) and short QT syndrome (see Chapter 2).

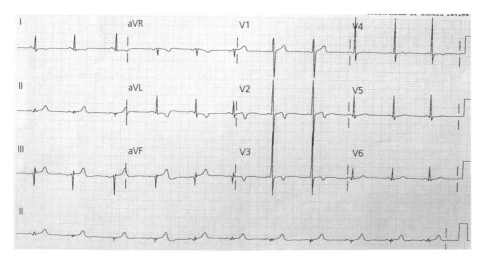

Figure 20.1 ECG showing abnormalities due to HCM.

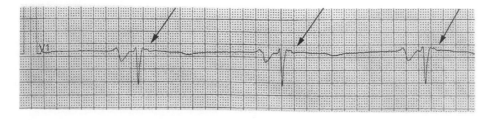

Figure 20.2 Rhythm strip showing presence of epsilon waves (arrowed).

Heat stroke

This is defined as a core temperature >40.6 °C and in athletes typically occurs during strenuous physical exercise (exertional heat stroke) when the environmental temperature and humidity are high. It may be exacerbated by the presence of hyperthyroidism, phaeochromocytoma or certain drugs, particularly sympathomimetics (e.g. cocaine).

Role of automated external defibrillators

Whatever the underlying pathophysiology, almost all victims of SCD associated with sport will have an arrhythmia, either ventricular fibrillation (VF) or VT, as the initial event. Therefore rapid recognition of cardiac arrest and early defibrillation is paramount, as demonstrated in a study of 1710 American high schools with an automated external defibrillator (AED). Of these schools, 36 (2.1%) reported a cardiac arrest, of which 14 arrests were in students (mean age 14 years, range 14–17 years), and 22 in non-students (mean age 57 years, range 42–71 years). Of the 36 cardiac arrests, 35 were witnessed and 34 received bystander CPR; 30 victims were defibrillated and 9/14 (64%) students survived, and 14/22 (64%) non-students survived. Despite nearly two-thirds of students surviving, this is probably less than might be anticipated following a witnessed collapse, bystander CPR and prompt defibrillation in a group of previously fit athletes.

One of the biggest obstacles to starting resuscitation seems to be the refusal to accept, by other participants and onlookers, that an apparently young, fit athlete has had a cardiac arrest. This frequently leads to delays in starting CPR and summoning and using a defibrillator.

Initial management of a collapsed athlete due to presumed cardiac cause

1 Rapidly confirm cardiac arrest – do not assume victim has fainted or been rendered unconscious.
2 At the same time:

Call for help, use a mobile phone to summon an ambulance
Send for AED if available.
Start CPR

3 Follow AED algorithm and continue CPR until help arrives.

Other points:
 – If the victim has been involved in a contact sport or there are any concerns about the victim's cervical spine, use the jaw thrust manoeuvre to open the airway, not a head tilt.
 – If heat stroke is suspected, standard protocols should be used with concurrent attempts to cool the victim using application of ice packs in the groins and axillae.

Cardiac arrest associated with trauma in sport

Trauma causing cardiac arrest has a high mortality with only around 5% of victims surviving; within this group the incidence of neurological disability is high. The common causes of cardiac arrest

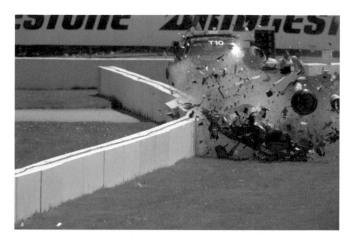

Figure 20.3 The mortality rate following traumatic cardiac arrest is very high. Vastly improved safety has dramatically reduced major injuries in motor sport. Reproduced with kind permission of the FIA Institute for Motor Sport Safety and Sustainability.

in victims of trauma include severe brain injury, hypovolaemia due to blood loss (e.g. massive skeletal injury, injury to liver, spleen, heart or major vessels) and hypoxia (e.g. massive pulmonary contusion, tension pneumothorax). Most of these occur during participation in sports such as motor racing (Figure 20.3) or equestrianism.

Management of a cardiac arrest secondary to trauma

Most cardiac arrests are due to pulseless electrical activity rather than VF or VT. Therefore identification and treatment of reversible causes is paramount.

1 Effective airway management is essential to prevent hypoxaemia and secondary neurological injury. Tracheal intubation should be performed if rescuers have the necessary skills, otherwise use an alternative, for example laryngeal mask airway (LMA). Failure of both ventilation and intubation is an indication for performing a surgical airway.
2 Avoid excessive ventilation, this reduces cardiac output, particularly in the hypovolaemic patient by impeding venous return and also worsens outcome in patients with traumatic brain injury (TBI). A tension pneumothorax should be decompressed with a lateral or anterior thoracostomy. This is more effective than a needle thoracostomy and quicker than inserting a chest drain.
3 Obvious external haemorrhage should be stemmed using direct pressure. Recent evidence from battle casualties has demonstrated that the use of tourniquets to stop exsanguinating haemorrhage from limb injuries is both safe and effective when applied correctly. Do not delay transfer to hospital while trying to establish IV access and give intravenous fluids. Where there is ongoing haemorrhage, large volumes of fluid may actually increase bleeding. When ultrasound is available along with a trained operator, its use may help with the diagnosis of haemoperitoneum, cardiac tamponade, haemothorax and pneumothorax.

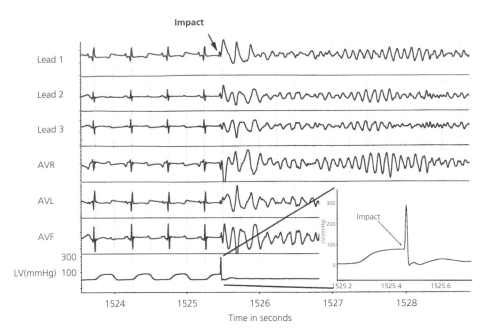

Figure 20.4 Animal model showing effect of precordial impact on intraventricular pressure and initiation of VF. Reprinted from Link MS, Maron BJ, VanderBrink BA, *et al*. *J Am Coll Cardiol*. 2001;37:649-54, Copyright © 2001, with permission from Elsevier.

Emergency thoracotomy is indicated on scene only when cardiac arrest is the result of penetrating chest trauma and the procedure can be performed within 10 minutes of the diagnosis of arrest. Within the emergency department, it is most effective when performed in those with penetrating cardiac injury who initially have signs of life and arrive with minimal delays. Up to 30% of these patients may survive. If the cause of the arrest is blunt trauma it should only be used in patients who arrest in the department; survival rates are poor, around 1.5%.

Key points:

- Survival is inversely related to on-scene time
- Treatment on scene should concentrate on high-quality CPR and exclusion of reversible causes
- Only undertake essential life-saving interventions, do not delay for spinal immobilisation

Commotio cordis

This is a rare cause of SCD, first described in the 1870s. When investigated in the 1930s, it was thought to be an 'exaggerated vagal reflex' causing the heart to stop. It follows a blunt, non-penetrating blow to the chest that causes VF and sudden death in the absence of any structural damage to the heart, ribs or sternum. The area of impact must be directly over precordium and occur 20 ms before the peak of the T wave. The impact results in a rapid rise in pressure activating ion channels and causing premature ventricular depolarisation which triggers VF (Figure 20.4). It is most common during organised or recreational sporting events, particularly ball games (Table 20.2), affecting young caucasian males (95%) with a mean age of 15 years. Its increasing recognition prompted the setting up of a National Commotio Cordis Registry in the USA in 1996.

Once again, a key issue is accepting that cardiac arrest has occurred in a previously well person, often of young age. Standard

Table 20.2 Causes of commotio cordis.

Equipment	Baseballs
	Softballs
	Hockey pucks
	Lacrosse ball
Physical contact	Knee, foot
	Elbow, forearm
	Fist
Recreational activities	Shadow boxing
	Kick from horse
	Gun recoil
	Bicycle handlebars

CPR guidelines should be followed, with the emphasis on early defibrillation as this is the only factor that has been shown to be associated with survival.

Summary

Cardiac arrest amongst competitors during sporting events is fortunately rare and most commonly has a cardiac cause; in the young it is usually a result of an underlying cardiac abnormality, while in the older athlete it is most commonly due to coronary artery disease. The mechanism of death in most cases is VF and therefore standard CPR guidelines should be followed. Unfortunately, outcomes are not as good as one might expect, most likely as a result of failure by bystanders to recognise and accept that cardiac arrest has occurred, resulting in a delay in treatment.

Further reading

Drezner JA. Preparing for sudden cardiac arrest – the essential role of automated external defibrillators in athletic medicine: a critical review. *Br J Sports Med* 2009;43:702–7.

Corrado D, Basso C, Pavel A, *et al.* Trends in sudden cardiovascular death in young athletes after implementation of a preparticipation screening program. *JAMA* 2006;**296**:1593–601.

Corrado D, Pelliccia A, Heidbuchel H, *et al.* Recommendations for interpretation of 12-lead electrocardiogram in the athlete. *Eur Heart J* 2010;**31**:243–59.

Drezner JA, Rao AL, Heistand J, Bloomingdale MK, Harmon KG. Effectiveness of emergency response planning for sudden cardiac arrest in United States high schools with automated external defibrillators. *Circulation* 2009;**120**:518–25.

Davies GE, Lockey DJ. Thirteen survivors of prehospital thoracotomy for penetrating trauma: a prehospital physician-performed resuscitation procedure that can yield good results. *J Trauma* 2011;**70**:E75–8.

Link MS, Maron BJ, VanderBrink BA, *et al.* Impact directly over the cardiac silhouette is necessary to produce ventricular fibrillation in an experimental model of commotio cordis. *J Am Coll Cardiol* 2001;**37**:649–54.

Maron BJ, Estes NAM. Commotio cordis. *N Engl J Med* 2010;**362**:917–27.

CHAPTER 21

Improving Outcomes from Cardiac Arrest: Quality, Education and Implementation

Jasmeet Soar[1] and Keith Couper[2]

[1]Southmead Hospital, North Bristol NHS Trust, Bristol, UK
[2]Heart of England NHS Foundation Trust, Birmingham, UK

OVERVIEW

- Delivering high-quality CPR requires interventions at a national, local, team and individual rescuer level
- Data from national registries, patient safety incident reports and mock-codes can be used to identify areas for improved practice
- Resuscitation team performance can be improved by ensuring teams brief and plan beforehand and also debrief using data collected during resuscitation events

---

Table 21.1 Aims of high-quality care.

Safe	Avoiding harm
Effective	Evidence based
Patient centred	Respectful care based on patient preferences, needs and values
Timely	Avoiding delays
Efficient	Avoiding waste
Equitable	Care quality does not vary according to issues such as race or socioeconomic status

Data from Committee on Quality of Health Care in America, Institute of Medicine. Crossing the Quality Chasm: A New Health System for the 21st Century, 2001.

Introduction

Improving outcomes from cardiac arrest requires high-quality care. Studies of both in- and out-of-hospital cardiac arrest show that there is a gap between what the guidelines say and what actually happens in clinical practice. The aims of high-quality care defined by the Institute of Medicine are that care has to be safe, effective, patient-centred, timely, efficient and equitable (Table 21.1). To achieve these aims, cardiac arrest care requires interventions at an international, national, local, team and individual rescuer level (Figure 21.1).

Measuring patient outcomes

Continuous measurement of compliance with processes, and patient outcomes at a national and local level provides information on the impact of changes in practice, identifies areas for improvement, and also enables comparison in outcomes between different organisations. The Utstein style provides standardised definitions and reporting templates for cardiac arrest processes (Figure 21.2).

Several registries and epidemiological databases already exist and the number is rapidly increasing (Table 21.2). Specifically, at a local level, registries allow participating organisations to track their progress over time to assess whether they are improving and also how they compare with similar organisations. A network of organisations that has an infrastructure to reliably collect data in standardized manner also enables the conduct of large multi-centre research studies.

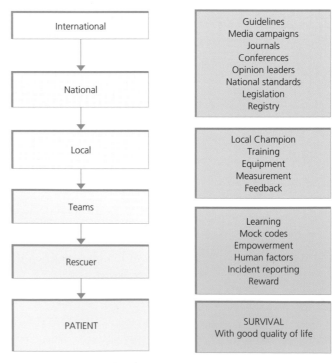

Figure 21.1 Examples of quality improvement interventions.

The quality of life in those who survive to leave hospital seems to be good, but survivors can have ongoing, physical, psychiatric and cognitive problems. There is currently no consensus on the best way of assessing long-term outcomes in cardiac arrest survivors. The Cerebral Performance Category (CPC) score is most

ABC of Resuscitation, Sixth Edition. Edited by Jasmeet Soar, Gavin D. Perkins and Jerry Nolan.
© 2013 John Wiley & Sons, Ltd. Published 2013 by John Wiley & Sons, Ltd.

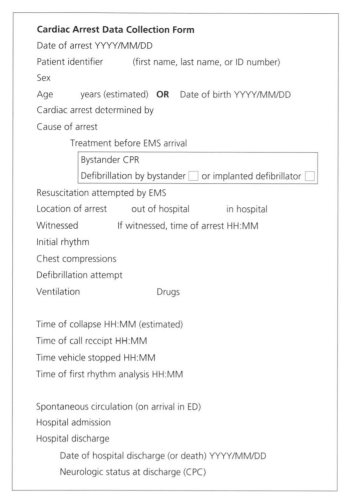

Cardiac Arrest Data Collection Form

Date of arrest YYYY/MM/DD

Patient identifier   (first name, last name, or ID number)

Sex

Age   years (estimated) **OR**   Date of birth YYYY/MM/DD

Cardiac arrest determined by

Cause of arrest

      Treatment before EMS arrival

        Bystander CPR

        Defibrillation by bystander ☐ or implanted defibrillator ☐

Resuscitation attempted by EMS

Location of arrest   out of hospital   in hospital

Witnessed   If witnessed, time of arrest HH:MM

Initial rhythm

Chest compressions

Defibrillation attempt

Ventilation   Drugs

Time of collapse HH:MM (estimated)

Time of call receipt HH:MM

Time vehicle stopped HH:MM

Time of first rhythm analysis HH:MM

Spontaneous circulation (on arrival in ED)

Hospital admission

Hospital discharge

      Date of hospital discharge (or death) YYYY/MM/DD

      Neurologic status at discharge (CPC)

Figure 21.2 A sample out-of hospital data collection form based on Utstein.

commonly used (Table 21.3). Survivors with a CPC score of 1 or 2 are usually said to have had a good neurological outcome. The CPC score is too crude, however, to describe more subtle problems that can occur in survivors.

Patient safety incident reporting

Studies show that clinical staff and, in particular, doctors rarely report safety incidents.

Incident reports are important as they can help identify problems with implementation and areas for improvement both locally and at higher levels. Safety incidents or errors reported during CPR are associated with a decrease in survival from cardiac arrest. The most commonly reported errors to the US Get With The Guidelines registry were related to giving drugs, defibrillation, airway management and chest compressions. Reports to the Danish Patient Safety Database have identified problems with alerting the resuscitation team, human performance, missing or failing equipment and medication errors.

Education and implementation

Survival from cardiac arrest is determined by the effectiveness of education and resources for implementation. The complexity of

Table 21.2 Examples of cardiac arrest registries and epidemiological databases and some key findings.

Details	In- or out-of hospital	Example of observations
American Heart Association Get With The Guidelines www.nrcpr.org Established 2000	In-hospital	In-hospital cardiac arrest survival data for adults and children Observation that worse survival at night and weekends Racial differences in survival after cardiac arrest
CARES (Cardiac Arrest Registry to Enhance Survival) www.cdc.gov/dhdsp /cares.htm Established 2004	Out-of-hospital	Outcome data Practice variation amongst emergency medicine systems
ROC (Resuscitation Outcomes Consortium Epistry) https://roc.uwctc.org /tiki/roc-public-home Established 2005	Out-of-hospital cardiac arrest	Clinical trial network Variation in outcomes Effect of CPR-quality on outcomes Interventional studies
NCAA (National Cardiac Arrest Audit) https://ncaa.icnarc.org Established 2009	In-hospital	Outcome data Comparative data Risk modelling

Table 21.3 The Cerebral Performance Category (CPC) score.

CPC	Definition
1	Good cerebral performance: conscious, alert, able to work, might have mild neurologic or psychological deficit
2	Moderate cerebral disability: conscious, sufficient cerebral function for independent activities of daily life. Able to work in sheltered environment
3	Severe cerebral disability: conscious, dependent on others for daily support because of impaired brain function. Ranges from ambulatory state to severe dementia or paralysis
4	Coma or vegetative state: any degree of coma without the presence of all brain death criteria. Unawareness, even if appears awake
5	Brain death: apnoea, areflexia, EEG silence, etc.

Based on Safar P. Resuscitation after Brain Ischemia In Grenvik A and Safar P (eds), *Brain Failure and Resuscitation*, pp. 155–84, Churchill Livingstone, New York, 1981.

educational interventions needs to be based on how many people need to learn the intervention, the complexity of the intervention and how often it will be used by the learner (Figure 21.3). Training has to be tailored to meet the needs of different groups. Ideally all citizens should know how to do CPR. This will range from training lay people who will rarely need to do CPR, non-healthcare staff who work in roles that mean they have a duty of care (e.g. lifeguards) and healthcare staff. Even amongst healthcare staff, the level of training will vary according to their role – those involved in acute emergency care are most likely to deal with cardiac arrests.

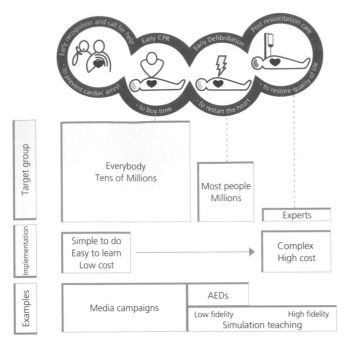

Figure 21.3 Implementing the chain of survival.

Numerous life support courses are available (see www.resus.org.uk). In the rest of this chapter we will discuss some emerging issues.

Compression-only CPR

Currently, only about a third of those who have an out-of-hospital cardiac arrest receive bystander CPR. To improve implementation, current guidelines suggest a staged approach:

- Ideally, full CPR skills (compressions and ventilation using a 30:2 ratio) should be taught to all citizens
- When training is time-limited or opportunistic, training should focus on chest compression-only CPR. An example is the British Heart Foundation 'Hands-only CPR campaign' (http://www.youtube.com/watch?v=ILxjxfB4zNk). This campaign has reached several million viewers and encouraged numerous individuals to get further training

- Ambulance dispatchers should provide guidance on compression-only CPR for primary cardiac arrest in adults
- For those trained in compression-only CPR, subsequent training should include training in ventilation as well as chest compressions
- Those laypersons with a duty of care, such as first aid workers, lifeguards and child minders, should be taught how to do chest compressions and ventilations
- If a child requires CPR, rescuers should be encouraged to use whichever adult sequence they have been taught, as outcome is worse if they do nothing. Non-specialists who wish to learn paediatric resuscitation because they have responsibility for children (e.g. parents, teachers, school nurses, lifeguards), should be taught that it is preferable to modify adult basic life support and give five initial breaths followed by approximately 1 minute of CPR before they go for help, if there is no-one to go for them. Chest compression depth for children is at least one-third of the anterior-posterior diameter of the chest

A new concept that helps those who rarely have to do CPR is 'just-in-time training'. One example is the use of automated external defibrillators (AEDs). Individuals should ideally train to use an AED, but if an untrained individual switches an AED on and follows the audiovisual prompts, they can save a life.

Checklists

Advanced level training is usually for healthcare providers. Checklists can be used to improve adherence to guidelines as long as they do not cause delays in starting CPR and the correct checklist is used. One example is the iResus smartphone application (Figure 21.4). This provides the guidelines in a step-by-step manner on a smartphone screen.

Mock codes

Mock cardiac arrest codes and drills using manikins or actors can be used to test the individual and system responses to cardiac arrest. For example, in the hospital setting, they can test the system to call for help, the resuscitation team response, the availability and function of equipment, and actual team performance. Mock codes

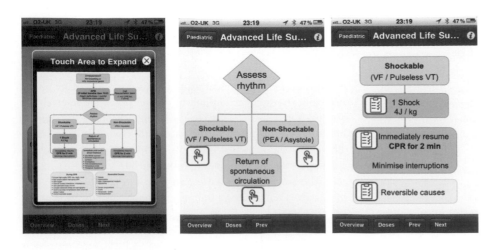

Figure 21.4 iResus smartphone app – screenshots. Reproduced with the kind permission of the Resuscitation Council (UK).

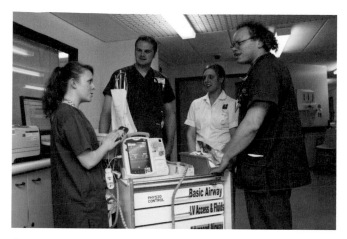

Figure 21.5 'Hot debriefing' with resuscitation team.

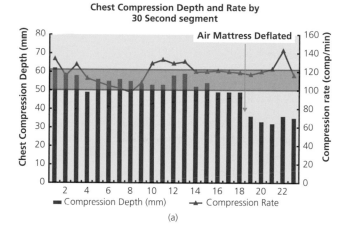

(a)

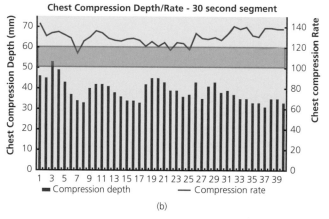

(b)

Figure 21.6 Example slides from a 'cold debriefing'.

can improve knowledge, skill performance, confidence, familiarity with the environment and identify system and user errors. An important aspect of any resuscitation attempt, whether it is actual or simulated, is debriefing individuals and the team.

Post-event debriefing

Post-event debriefing can improve individual and team cardiac arrest performance. Post-event debriefing involves a facilitated discussion, where team members are encouraged to discuss issues and identify strategies for improvement. The focus should be education and quality improvement; issues of blame must be avoided for the process to work effectively. Post-event debriefing may occur either immediately following the event ('hot' debriefing) or may be delayed ('cold' debriefing); each format has specific advantages and difficulties.

'Hot' post-event debriefing

Hot debriefings are normally led by the resuscitation team leader, focus on immediate issues and concerns, and are usually of short duration (Figure 21.5). This can be difficult if the patient has a return of spontaneous circulation, as focus then inevitably shifts to post-resuscitation care. Where the cardiac arrest has been particularly difficult or involved junior staff, hot post-event debriefing can have psychological benefits.

'Cold' post-event debriefing

A facilitator who was not a resuscitation team member normally leads cold post-event debriefings. They work most effectively when discussion is based on objective data, such as CPR performance data, observation or video recording (Figure 21.6). Cold debriefings will typically be longer (up to 30 minutes). The debrief should be sufficiently timely to ensure team members have good event recollection, although a key difficulty with this approach is identifying a meeting time that all team members can attend.

Further reading

Committee on Quality of Health Care in America, Institute of Medicine. *Crossing the Quality Chasm: A New Health System for the 21st Century*. Washington, DC: The National Academies Press, 2001.

Edelson DP, Litzinger B, Arora V, *et al*. Improving in-hospital cardiac arrest process and outcomes with performance debriefing. *Arch Intern Med* 2008;**168**(10):1063–9.

Elliott VJ, Rodgers DL, Brett SJ. Systematic review of quality of life and other patient-centred outcomes after cardiac arrest survival. *Resuscitation* 2011;**82**(3):247–56.

Jacobs I, Nadkarni V, Bahr J, *et al*. Cardiac arrest and cardiopulmonary resuscitation outcome reports: update and simplification of the Utstein templates for resuscitation registries. A statement for healthcare professionals from a task force of the International Liaison Committee on Resuscitation (American Heart Association, European Resuscitation Council, Australian Resuscitation Council, New Zealand Resuscitation Council, Heart and Stroke Foundation of Canada, InterAmerican Heart Foundation, Resuscitation Council of Southern Africa). *Resuscitation* 2004;**63**(3):233–49.

Ornato JP, Peberdy MA, Reid RD, Feeser VR, Dhindsa HS. NRCPR Investigators. Impact of resuscitation system errors on survival from in-hospital cardiac arrest. *Resuscitation* 2012;**83**(1):63–9.

Safar P. Resuscitation after brain ischemia. In Grenvik A and Safar P (eds), *Brain Failure and Resuscitation*, pp. 155–184. Churchill Livingstone, New York, 1981.

Soar J, Edelson DP, Perkins GD. Delivering high-quality cardiopulmonary resuscitation in-hospital. *Curr Opin Crit Care* 2011;**17**(3):225–30.

CHAPTER 22

Decisions Relating to Resuscitation

Serena Cottrell[1] and David Pitcher[2]

[1]Queen Alexandra Hospital, Portsmouth, UK
[2]University Hospital Birmingham, Worcester, UK

OVERVIEW

- The ethical framework for resuscitation decisions requires consideration of autonomy, beneficence, non-maleficence and justice or equality
- Do not attempt cardiopulmonary resuscitation (DNACPR) decisions are appropriate if attempting CPR would be futile, if the patient refuses CPR or attempting CPR would not lead to overall benefit for the patient
- Communicating with patients and those close to them about DNACPR decisions is essential
- Clear systems should be in place to ensure that DNACPR decisions are communicated effectively amongst the healthcare team and between different healthcare settings

Introduction

Deciding whether or not it is appropriate to attempt cardiopulmonary resuscitation (CPR) often evokes strong emotions in patients and their families and within the multidisciplinary team. When there is any element of doubt, the default position in most healthcare settings is to attempt to preserve life, although this has been questioned; some clinicians have suggested that there should be an opt-in policy for CPR. This chapter focuses on the ethical aspects of the decision-making process and the importance of effective communication. However, it is crucial that all such decisions are made within the law of the appropriate country or state. For illustration purposes, reference will be made in this chapter to some aspects of the law that applies in England and Wales (e.g. The Mental Capacity Act 2005). Healthcare professionals have a responsibility to be aware of the law that applies in their place of practice; there are differences in some aspects of the law in other parts of the UK and in other countries.

For the purposes of this chapter the terminology used for a decision not to attempt CPR will be DNACPR (Do not attempt cardiopulmonary resuscitation). Box 22.1 illustrates the range of terminology that can be found.

ABC of Resuscitation, Sixth Edition. Edited by Jasmeet Soar, Gavin D. Perkins and Jerry Nolan.
© 2013 John Wiley & Sons, Ltd. Published 2013 by John Wiley & Sons, Ltd.

Box 22.1 **Terminology**

- DNR (Do not resuscitate)
- DNAR (Do not attempt resuscitation)
- DNACPR (Do not attempt cardiopulmonary resuscitation)

Ethical principles

There are considered to be four key principles related to medical ethics decision-making in addition to sanctity-of-life doctrine. These are shown in Box 22.2.

Box 22.2 **Ethical principles**

- Autonomy (self-determination that is free from controlling interferences by others preventing meaningful choice)
- Beneficence (acting in the person's best interests)
- Non-maleficence (doing no harm)
- Justice or equality

Autonomy is a key principle for DNACPR decisions. If an adult (a person aged 18 years or above) chooses to refuse CPR and is considered to have capacity for that decision, their view must be respected even if it appears extreme. If an adult is not able to make a decision, for example when they are unconscious, then the decision maker still needs to consider any previously expressed views. An example of this is an Advance Decision, which gives an adult the opportunity to record their wishes regarding their future care in case they become unable to make decisions for themselves and may include a statement refusing resuscitation. This document is legally binding in England and Wales but must be signed and witnessed and state specifically that it should apply even if their life is at stake.

Another way that people have tried to inform others of their wishes regarding CPR is to have a 'Do not Resuscitate' tattoo. From an ethical and legal point of view this presents difficulties as it is impossible to know whether this tattoo represents a valid advance decision at the time of a cardiac arrest. The person may have changed their mind or the decision may be based on a prognosis that is out of date. Additionally patients and the public may not always have a clear or realistic understanding of their diagnosis or the benefits, burdens and risks of CPR, as the public's knowledge about the clinical complexities may be limited (General Medical Council (GMC) Guidance 2010).

Applying ethical principles

Balancing the principles of beneficence and non-maleficence and helping people to understand that balance in using their autonomy to make decisions is often difficult. Bringing someone back to life from cardiorespiratory arrest is clearly in their best interests if they recover to a quality and duration of life that they regard as worthwhile, whereas resuscitating someone who then has to endure severe disability or suffering and a quality of life that they find intolerable has done more harm than good. In helping patients and those close to them with CPR decisions, it is crucial to explain the potential risks associated with CPR as well as the possible benefit, and the lack of certainty about the outcome. Finally to incorporate justice and equality in CPR decisions it is important to ensure that these decisions are not influenced by factors such as age, gender, race or religious beliefs. Of these, perhaps age is the most challenging but rigorous attention to the other three principles, irrespective of age, will help to ensure that appropriate decisions are made.

When are decisions about CPR appropriate?

Planning in advance for anyone at risk of a cardiorespiratory arrest (e.g. those with life-limiting or life-threatening disease) is an important part of clinical care. This should include decisions about CPR (Joint statement by the British Medical Association (BMA), Resuscitation Council (UK) (RCUK) and the Royal College of Nursing (RCN) 2007) as well as other palliative care decisions such as symptom control and psychological, cultural and spiritual wishes. This is relevant for many people in the community as well as those admitted to hospitals and other healthcare institutions.

A decision not to attempt CPR may be considered in three broad sets of circumstances as shown in Box 22.3.

Box 22.3 **Circumstances in which a DNACPR order may be appropriate**

- CPR will not re-start the heart and breathing
- CPR is refused by a patient with capacity or there is a valid Advance Decision in a patient who lacks capacity
- CPR is considered not to be in the patient's best interests as the risks of CPR outweigh the benefits

When CPR will not re-start the heart

CPR will not be successful in re-starting the heart and breathing if a cardiorespiratory arrest is part of the dying process in a terminal condition and so should not be attempted. CPR in these circumstances will result in a loss of dignity and hinder a good death. The term medical futility has been used to describe this situation; however 'futility' is open to a number of subjective interpretations and so is probably best avoided.

Refusal of CPR

This arises when, irrespective of the likelihood of successful resuscitation, the person chooses to refuse CPR. In the case of a person without capacity, that refusal would have to have been recorded as a valid Advance Decision to refuse treatment. To be valid, an Advance Decision must apply in the specific circumstances present at the time of the event. For example, it would be appropriate to provide immediate treatment to relieve airway obstruction due to choking, if this situation had not been foreseen and specified in the Advance Decision.

There may also be situations where suspension of a DNACPR decision (including an Advance Decision) requires careful consideration. This may become appropriate when a patient is undergoing a procedure such as cardiac catheterisation or a surgical operation and the chances of immediate, effective treatment of cardiorespiratory arrest are high. The Royal College of Anaesthetists advises that all DNACPR orders should be reconsidered in these circumstances, and decisions made about what resuscitation is appropriate for each individual, including CPR. Once again, autonomy must be paramount in these decisions, and some patients with an Advance Decision will want it to remain in force in these circumstances. Box 22.4 describes situations when a review of the CPR decision may be appropriate.

Box 22.4 **Review of DNACPR decisions**

It is important to review the appropriateness of every DNACPR decision whenever:

- the patient's clinical condition changes
- review is requested by the patient, those close to them, or by a member of the multidisciplinary team
- the patient moves to a different healthcare setting

Cancellation of a DNACPR decision may be appropriate if the patient's clinical condition improves, making the chances of a successful outcome from CPR much greater than it had been

When CPR is considered not to be in the person's best interests

This occurs when the risks of CPR are considered to outweigh the benefits. These are often the most challenging decisions of the three situations. In this situation it is important to involve the patient in the decision whenever possible, and to ensure that they are given adequate information to make an informed decision. Even if there is only a small chance that resuscitation will be successful and a person decides that they wish to receive CPR, this should not be denied on the grounds of the healthcare professional's perceived potential for that person to experience excessive suffering or poor quality of life.

Communication

Good communication is a crucial part of good medical practice, no more so than in discussions about CPR. Discussions about the appropriateness of CPR may need several conversations over a period of time and ideally are undertaken by the clinician who knows the patient best. This is particularly relevant when the CPR decision involves a child or young person whose ability to contribute to the discussion may change over a relatively short period of time. It is important that those initiating CPR discussions ensure that the patient does not feel rushed and is given plenty of opportunity to ask questions and also given information on who to contact should more questions arise.

Communication may be aided by the use of patient information leaflets which should include instruction on who to approach if there should be a change of mind about CPR (Figures 22.1 and 22.2). However, information leaflets should be used to support and supplement sensitive discussions with patients and those close to them and should never be used as an alternative to spending adequate time undertaking such individual discussions.

There are several important aspects of communication that apply to CPR decisions (Boxes 22.5 and 22.6). It is very important to communicate with the patient, provided they have capacity. Communication with those close to the patient is also important, whilst at the same time respecting the patient's wishes with regard to confidentiality. Some people may choose to keep a terminal diagnosis and/or a DNACPR decision from those close to them, so in a patient with capacity their consent must be obtained before discussion with their family or friends.

Information for you,
your relatives and carers about
Do Not Attempt
Cardiopulmonary Resuscitation
decisions

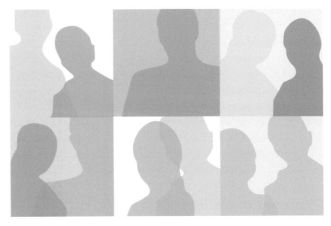

Figure 22.1 Example of information leaflet for patients, relatives and carers.

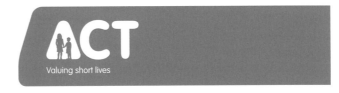

Box 22.5 **Starting the conversation**

- It is always important when discussing decisions about CPR that a healthcare professional has clear in their mind the purpose of the discussion before sitting down with the patient and/or their family
- If a DNACPR decision has been made on medical grounds, because cardiorespiratory arrest would be part of the process of death in a terminal condition and CPR would not be successful, the purpose of the meeting is to inform the patient or their family of the decision and the reasons for it
- If the balance of risk and benefit from CPR is less certain, the purpose will be to explain the risks and benefits and explore the patient's wishes in order to facilitate an informed decision

---

A parent's guide:
Making critical care
choices for your child

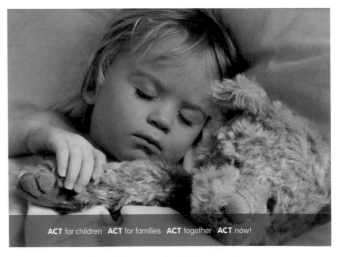

Box 22.6 **Communication pitfalls**

- Failure to communicate effectively with patients and their families is the most common cause of complaints about DNACPR decisions
- It is better to have told a patient about a decision that has been made and the reasons for it than to have them find out by chance and possibly misunderstand
- In law doctors are not required to give treatment that they believe to be inappropriate, so patients may not insist on receiving CPR if the doctor treating them recommends otherwise

In reality if there is disagreement such that a patient believes that they should be offered CPR and their doctor does not, it is best to seek a second opinion

---

Figure 22.2 Example of information leaflet for parents.

Communicating with those close to the patient

If a person lacks capacity (Box 22.7), those close to them should be involved in discussions to explore their wishes, feelings, beliefs and values. It is important that all such discussions are undertaken

Box 22.7 **Test of capacity**

Definition

A person lacks capacity if they have an impairment or disturbance that affects the way their mind or brain works and the impairment or disturbance means that they are unable to make a specific decision at the time that it needs to be made

This test should be used if a clinician has cause to believe a person lacks capacity

A person is deemed to be 'unable to make a decision' if they cannot:

- understand information relating to the decision that has to be made, or
- retain that information in their mind for the duration of the conversation, or
- use or weigh that information as part of the decision-making process, or
- communicate their decision

DO NOT ATTEMPT CARDIOPULMONARY RESUSCITATION

Adults aged 16 years and over

DNARadult.1(March 2009)

Name _____

Address _____

Date of birth _____

NHS or hospital number _____

Date of DNAR order:

/ /

DO NOT PHOTOCOPY

In the event of cardiac or respiratory arrest no attempts at cardiopulmonary resuscitation (CPR) will be made. All other appropriate treatment and care will be provided.

1 | Does the patient have capacity to make and communicate decisions about CPR? If "YES" go to box 2 — YES / NO

If "NO", are you aware of a valid advance decision refusing CPR which is relevant to the current condition?" If "YES" go to box 6 — YES / NO

If "NO", has the patient appointed a Welfare Attorney to make decisions on their behalf? If "YES" they must be consulted. — YES / NO

All other decisions must be made in the patient's best interests and comply with current law. Go to box 2

2 | Summary of the main clinical problems and reasons why CPR would be inappropriate, unsuccessful or not in the patient's best interests:

3 | Summary of communication with patient (or Welfare Attorney). If this decision has not been discussed with the patient or Welfare Attorney state the reason why:

4 | Summary of communication with patient's relatives or friends:

5 | Names of members of multidisciplinary team contributing to this decision:

6 | Healthcare professional completing this DNAR order:

Name _____ Position _____

Signature _____ Date _____ Time _____

7 | Review and endorsement by most senior health professional:

Signature _____ Name _____ Date _____

Review date (if appropriate)

Signature _____ Name _____ Date _____

Signature _____ Name _____ Date _____

Figure 22.3 Resuscitation Council (UK) model form for adults, for use in England and Wales.

with sensitivity and with clarity, by a professional trained and experienced in doing this. Those close to the person must not be made to feel that *they* are making a decision; they are simply providing valuable information to enable the healthcare team to make a decision in the best interests of the patient.

Communication between healthcare professionals

Communication between healthcare professionals is also crucial to the effective use of CPR decisions. When someone suffers cardiorespiratory arrest, CPR should be started immediately. If a DNACPR decision has been made, it is important that all the professionals involved in the patient's care are aware of or have immediate access to that decision and its current validity at the time of a cardiorespiratory arrest, so that CPR is not started in error. Good handover of information between staff and clear recording of the decision in an immediately available location are essential. The Resuscitation Council (UK) recommends the use of a standard form for recording DNACPR decisions and the basis for them, so that its appearance and content are familiar to all healthcare staff (Figures 22.3 and 22.4). If CPR has been started in a patient and a valid Advance Decision or DNACPR decision is then located, it is appropriate to cease further resuscitation attempts. For a DNACPR order to be maximally effective, it must travel with the patient, in the community, within a hospital or other institution and during transfers, for example by ambulance. This becomes more difficult if the patient has not been made aware of the DNACPR decision.

Figure 22.4 Resuscitation Council (UK) model form for children under 16 years, for use in England and Wales.

The increasing use of paperless, electronic patient records in both primary care and hospitals will present new challenges in our efforts to ensure that DNACPR decisions are accessible immediately when they are needed. However, electronic records could be constructed to help clinicians to achieve better documentation of the reasons for the decision and the discussions that have occurred.

Further reading

Beauchamp T, *Childress J. Principles of Biomedical Ethics.* Oxford University Press, 2009.

British Medical Association, The Resuscitation Council (UK) and the Royal College of Nursing. Decisions relating to cardiopulmonary resuscitation. A joint statement. October 2007. www.resus.org.uk.

General Medical Council. Treatment and care towards the end of life: good practice in decision making. http://www.gmc-uk.org/guidance/ethical_guidance/end_of_life_care.asp. 2010.

NHS End-of-Life Care Programme and The National Council for Palliative Care. Advance Decision to refuse Treatment, a guide for health and social care professionals. London, Department of Health, 2008.

Royal College of Physicians. *Advance Care Planning.* London, Royal College of Physicians, 2009.

Sokol D.K, Mc Fadzean W.A, Dickson W.A, Whitaker I.S. Ethical dilemmas in the acute setting. *BMJ* 2011:**343**:d5528.

Index

Note: Page references in *italics* refer to Figures; those in **bold** refer to Tables

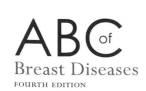

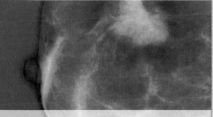

ABC of Breast Diseases

4TH EDITION

J. Michael Dixon
Western General Hospital, Edinburgh, UK

Breast diseases are common and often encountered by health professionals in primary care. While the incidence of breast cancer is increasing, earlier detection and improved treatments are helping to reduce breast cancer mortality. The *ABC of Breast Diseases, 4th Edition*:

- Provides comprehensive guidance to the assessment of symptoms, how to manage common breast conditions and guidelines on referral
- Covers congenital problems, breast infection and mastalgia, before addressing the epidemiology, prevention, screening and diagnosis of breast cancer and outlines the treatment and management options for breast cancer within different groups
- Includes new chapters on the genetics, prevention, management of high risk women and the psychological aspects of breast diseases
- Is ideal for GPs, family physicians, practice nurses and breast care nurses as well as for surgeons and oncologists both in training and recently qualified as well as medical students

AUGUST 2012 | 9781444337969 | 168 PAGES | £27.99/US$46.95/€35.90/AU$52.95

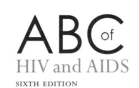

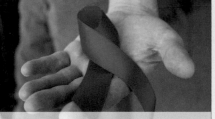

ABC of HIV and AIDS

6TH EDITION

Michael W. Adler, Simon G. Edwards, Robert F. Miller, Gulshan Sethi & Ian Williams
University College London Medical School; Mortimer Market Centre, London; University College London; St Thomas' Hospital, London Medical School; University College London Medical School

Since the previous edition, big advances have been made in treatment, knowledge of the disease and epidemiology. The problem of AIDS in developing countries has become a major political and humanitarian issue.

- Edited by the Director of the Department for Sexually Transmitted Diseases, *ABC of HIV and AIDS, 6th Edition* is an authoritative guide to the epidemiology, incidence, and most up to date management of HIV and AIDS
- Reflects the constantly changing knowledge of the disease and its manifestations, new developments in drug and non-drug management, sociological and political issues
- Includes 6 new chapters on conditions associated with AIDS and further concentration on the community effects of the disease, and the situation of women with AIDS
- Ideal for all levels of health care workers caring for HIV and AIDS patients

JUNE 2012 | 9781405157001 | 144 PAGES | £24.99/US$49.95/€32.90/AU$47.95

ABC of Pain
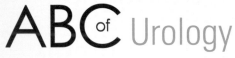

Lesley A. Colvin & Marie Fallon
Western General Hospital, Edinburgh; University of Edinburgh

Pain is a common presentation and this brand new title focuses on the pain management issues most often encountered in primary care. *ABC of Pain*:

- Covers all the chronic pain presentations in primary care right through to tertiary and palliative care and includes guidance on pain management in special groups such as pregnancy, children, the elderly and the terminally ill
- Includes new findings on the effectiveness of interventions and the progression to acute pain and appropriate pharmacological management
- Features pain assessment, epidemiology and the evidence base in a truly comprehensive reference
- Provides a global perspective with an international list of expert contributors

JUNE 2012 | 9781405176217 | 128 PAGES | £24.99/US$44.95/€32.90/AU$47.95

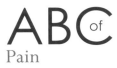
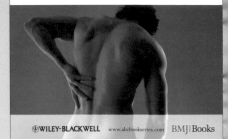

ABC of Urology
3RD EDITION

Chris Dawson & Janine Nethercliffe
Fitzwilliam Hospital, Peterborough; Edith Cavell Hospital, Peterborough

Urological conditions are common, accounting for up to one third of all surgical admissions to hospital. Outside of hospital care urological problems are a common reason for patients needing to see their GP.

- *ABC of Urology, 3rd Edition* provides a comprehensive overview of urology
- Focuses on the diagnosis and management of the most common urological conditions
- Features 4 additional chapters: improved coverage of renal and testis cancer in separate chapters and new chapters on management of haematuria, laparoscopy, trauma and new urological advances
- Ideal for GPs and trainee GPs, and is useful for junior doctors undergoing surgical training, while medical students and nurses undertaking a urological placement as part of their training programme will find this edition indispensable

MARCH 2012 | 9780470657171 | 88 PAGES | £23.99/US$37.95/€30.90/AU$47.95

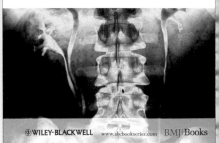

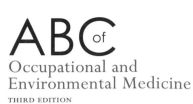

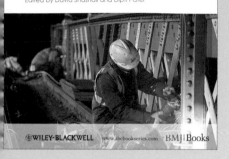

ABC of Occupational and Environmental Medicine

3RD EDITION

David Snashall & Dipti Patel

Guy's & St. Thomas' Hospital, London; Medical Advisory Service for Travellers Abroad (MASTA)

Since the publication of last edition, there have been huge changes in the world of occupational health. It has become firmly a part of international public health, and in Britain there is now a National Director for Work and Health. This fully updated new edition embraces these changes and:

- Provides comprehensive guidance on current occupational and environmental health practice and legislation
- Concentrates on the newer kinds of occupational disease, for example 'RSI', pesticide poisoning and electromagnetic radiation, where exposure and effects are difficult to understand
- Places an emphasis on work, health and well-being, and the public health benefits of work, the value of work, disabled people at work, the aging workforce, and vocational rehabilitation
- Includes chapters on the health effects of climate change and of occupational health and safety in relation to migration and terrorism

NOVEMBER 2012 | 9781444338171 | 168 PAGES | £27.99/US$44.95/€38.90/AU$52.95

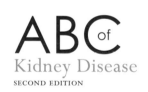

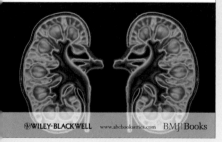

ABC of Kidney Disease

2ND EDITION

David Goldsmith, Satish Jayawardene & Penny Ackland

Guy's & St. Thomas' Hospital, London; King's College Hospital, London; Melbourne Grove Medical Practice, London

Nephrology is sometimes considered a complicated and specialized topic and the illustrative ABC format will help GPs quickly and easily assimilate the information needed. *ABC of Kidney Disease, 2nd Edition*:

- Is a practical guide to the most common renal diseases to enable non-renal health care workers to screen, identify, treat and refer renal patients appropriately and to provide the best possible care
- Covers organizational aspects of renal disease management, dialysis and transplantation
- Provides an explanatory glossary of renal terms, guidance on anaemia management and information on drug prescribing and interactions
- Has been fully revised in accordance with new guidelines

OCTOBER 2012 | 9780470672044 | 112 PAGES | £27.99/US$44.95/€35.90/AU$52.95

ALSO AVAILABLE

ABC of Adolescence
Russell Viner
2005 | 9780727915740 | 56 PAGES
£26.99 / US$41.95 / €34.90 / AU$52.95

ABC of Antithrombotic Therapy
Gregory Y. H. Lip & Andrew D. Blann
2003 | 9780727917713 | 67 PAGES
£26.50 / US$41.95 / €34.90 / AU$52.95

ABC of Arterial and Venous Disease, 2nd Edition
Richard Donnelly & Nick J. M. London
2009 | 9781405178891 | 120 PAGES
£31.50 / US$54.95 / €40.90 / AU$59.95

ABC of Asthma, 6th Edition
John Rees, Dipak Kanabar & Shriti Pattani
2009 | 9781405185967 | 104 PAGES
£26.99 / US$41.95 / €34.90 / AU$52.95

ABC of Burns
Shehan Hettiaratchy, Remo Papini & Peter Dziewulski
2004 | 9780727917874 | 56 PAGES
£26.50 / US$41.95 / €34.90 / AU$52.95

ABC of Child Protection, 4th Edition
Roy Meadow, Jacqueline Mok & Donna Rosenberg
2007 | 9780727918178 | 120 PAGES
£35.50 / US$59.95 / €45.90 / AU$67.95

ABC of Clinical Electrocardiography, 2nd Edition
Francis Morris, William J. Brady & John Camm
2008 | 9781405170642 | 112 PAGES
£34.50 / US$57.95 / €44.90 / AU$67.95

ABC of Clinical Genetics, 3rd Edition
Helen M. Kingston
2002 | 9780727916273 | 120 PAGES
£34.50 / US$57.95 / €44.90 / AU$67.95

ABC of Clinical Haematology, 3rd Edition
Drew Provan
2007 | 9781405153539 | 112 PAGES
£34.50 / US$59.95 / €44.90 / AU$67.95

ABC of Clinical Leadership
Tim Swanwick & Judy McKimm
2010 | 9781405198172 | 88 PAGES
£20.95 / US$32.95 / €26.90 / AU$39.95

ABC of Complementary Medicine, 2nd Edition
Catherine Zollman, Andrew J. Vickers & Janet Richardson
2008 | 9781405136570 | 64 PAGES
£28.95 / US$47.95 / €37.90 / AU$54.95

ABC of COPD, 2nd Edition
Graeme P. Currie
2010 | 9781444333886 | 88 PAGES
£23.95 / US$37.95 / €30.90 / AU$47.95

ABC of Dermatology, 5th Edition
Paul K. Buxton & Rachael Morris-Jones
2009 | 9781405170659 | 224 PAGES
£34.50 / US$58.95 / €44.90 / AU$67.95

ABC of Diabetes, 6th Edition
Tim Holt & Sudhesh Kumar
2007 | 9781405177849 | 112 PAGES
£31.50 / US$52.95 / €40.90 / AU$59.95

ABC of Eating Disorders
Jane Morris
2008 | 9780727918437 | 80 PAGES
£26.50 / US$41.95 / €34.90 / AU$52.95

ABC of Emergency Differential Diagnosis
Francis Morris & Alan Fletcher
2009 | 9781405170635 | 96 PAGES
£31.50 / US$55.95 / €40.90 / AU$59.95

ABC of Geriatric Medicine
Nicola Cooper, Kirsty Forrest & Graham Mulley
2009 | 9781405169424 | 88 PAGES
£26.50 / US$44.95 / €34.90 / AU$52.95

ABC of Headache
Anne MacGregor & Alison Frith
2008 | 9781405170666 | 88 PAGES
£23.95 / US$41.95 / €30.90 / AU$47.95

ABC of Heart Failure, 2nd Edition
Russell C. Davis, Michael K. Davis & Gregory Y. H. Lip
2006 | 9780727916440 | 72 PAGES
£26.50 / US$41.95 / €34.90 / AU$52.95

ABC of Imaging in Trauma
Leonard J. King & David C. Wherry
2008 | 9781405183321 | 144 PAGES
£31.50 / US$50.95 / €40.90 / AU$59.95

ABC of Interventional Cardiology, 2nd Edition
Ever D. Grech
2010 | 9781405170673 | 120 PAGES
£25.95 / US$40.95 / €33.90 / AU$49.95

ABC of Learning and Teaching in Medicine, 2nd Edition
Peter Cantillon & Diana Wood
2009 | 9781405185974 | 96 PAGES
£22.99 / US$35.95 / €29.90 / AU$44.95

ABC of Liver, Pancreas and Gall Bladder
Ian Beckingham
1905 | 9780727915313 | 64 PAGES
£24.95 / US$39.95 / €32.90 / AU$47.95

ABC of Lung Cancer
Ian Hunt, Martin M. Muers & Tom Treasure
2009 | 9781405146524 | 64 PAGES
£25.95 / US$41.95 / €33.90 / AU$49.95

ABC of Medical Law
Lorraine Corfield, Ingrid Granne & William Latimer-Sayer
2009 | 9781405176286 | 64 PAGES
£24.95 / US$39.95 / €32.90 / AU$47.95

ABC of Mental Health, 2nd Edition
Teifion Davies & Tom Craig
2009 | 9780727916396 | 128 PAGES
£32.50 / US$52.95 / €41.90 / AU$62.95

ABC of Obesity
Naveed Sattar & Mike Lean
2007 | 9781405136747 | 64 PAGES
£24.99 / US$39.99 / €32.90 / AU$47.95

ABC of One to Seven, 5th Edition
Bernard Valman
2009 | 9781405181051 | 168 PAGES
£32.50 / US$52.95 / €41.90 / AU$62.95

ABC of Palliative Care, 2nd Edition
Marie Fallon & Geoffrey Hanks
2006 | 9781405130790 | 96 PAGES
£30.50 / US$52.95 / €39.90 / AU$57.95

ABC of Patient Safety
John Sandars & Gary Cook
2007 | 9781405156929 | 64 PAGES
£28.50 / US$46.99 / €36.90 / AU$54.95

ABC of Practical Procedures
Tim Nutbeam & Ron Daniels
2009 | 9781405185950 | 144 PAGES
£31.50 / US$50.95 / €40.90 / AU$59.95

ABC of Preterm Birth
William McGuire & Peter Fowlie
2005 | 9780727917638 | 56 PAGES
£26.50 / US$41.95 / €34.90 / AU$52.95

ABC of Psychological Medicine
Richard Mayou, Michael Sharpe & Alan Carson
2003 | 9780727915566 | 72 PAGES
£26.99 / US$41.95 / €34.90 / AU$52.95

ABC of Rheumatology, 4th Edition
Ade Adebajo
2009 | 9781405170680 | 192 PAGES
£31.95 / US$50.95 / €41.90 / AU$62.95

ABC of Sepsis
Ron Daniels & Tim Nutbeam
2009 | 9781405181945 | 104 PAGES
£31.50 / US$52.95 / €40.90 / AU$59.95

ABC of Sexual Health, 2nd Edition
John Tomlinson
2004 | 9780727917591 | 96 PAGES
£31.50 / US$52.95 / €40.90 / AU$59.95

ABC of Skin Cancer
Sajjad Rajpar & Jerry Marsden
2008 | 9781405162197 | 80 PAGES
£26.50 / US$47.95 / €34.90 / AU$52.95

ABC of Spinal Disorders
Andrew Clarke, Alwyn Jones & Michael O'Malley
2009 | 9781405170697 | 72 PAGES
£24.95 / US$39.95 / €32.90 / AU$47.95

ABC of Sports and Exercise Medicine, 3rd Edition
Gregory Whyte, Mark Harries & Clyde Williams
2005 | 9780727918130 | 136 PAGES
£34.95 / US$62.95 / €44.90 / AU$67.95

ABC of Subfertility
Peter Braude & Alison Taylor
2005 | 9780727915344 | 64 PAGES
£24.95 / US$39.95 / €32.90 / AU$47.95

ABC of the First Year, 6th Edition
Bernard Valman & Roslyn Thomas
2009 | 9781405180375 | 136 PAGES
£31.50 / US$55.95 / €40.90 / AU$59.95

ABC of the Upper Gastrointestinal Tract
Robert Logan, Adam Harris & J. J. Misiewicz
2002 | 9780727912664 | 54 PAGES
£26.50 / US$41.95 / €34.90 / AU$52.95

ABC of Transfusion, 4th Edition
Marcela Contreras
2009 | 9781405156462 | 128 PAGES
£31.50 / US$55.95 / €40.90 / AU$59.95

ABC of Tubes, Drains, Lines and Frames
Adam Brooks, Peter F. Mahoney & Brian Rowlands
2008 | 9781405160148 | 88 PAGES
£26.50 / US$41.95 / €34.90 / AU$52.95

For more information on any of our medical books, please visit **www.wiley.com/go/medicine**